The Sleep Book

The Sleep Book

How to Sleep Well Every Night

DR GUY MEADOWS

This edition first published in Great Britain in 2014 by
Orion
an imprint of the Orion Publishing Group Ltd
Orion House, 5 Upper St Martin's Lane,
London WC2H 9EA
An Hachette UK Company

1 3 5 7 9 10 8 6 4 2

A CIP catalogue record for this book is available
from the British Library.

Trade Paperback ISBN: 978 1 409 14910 1

Illustrations and cover illustration by Pola Gruszka.

Printed in Great Britain by CPI Group (UK) Ltd, Croydon CR0 4YY

The Orion Publishing Group's policy is to use papers that are natural,
renewable and recyclable and made from wood grown in sustainable
forests. The logging and manufacturing processes are expected to conform
to the environmental regulations of the country of origin.

Every effort has been made to fulfil requirements with regard to
reproducing copyright material. The author and publisher will be glad to
rectify any omissions at the earliest opportunity.

www.orionbooks.co.uk

While every effort has been made to ensure that the information in this
book is correct, it should not be taken as offering medical advice.
People under medical supervision should not adopt the programme,
or change or come off their medication without first speaking to
their GP and following their advice.

Acknowledgements

I would like to thank all my clients from whom I have learnt so much from over the years. My business partner Aid, for his inspiring work and tireless efforts in creating The Sleep School. Pola, for creating all the amazing illustrations and animations. Orion, for believing in the potential of this work – especially Jane, Emma and the rest of the team who have worked so hard. Jacq, for her fantastic editing. Everyone within the ACT community for pioneering such a fantastic therapy. My mother, for her continued support of my work, and to Angela, for her endless proofreading. Finally, a huge thank you to my wife Kathryn for her never-ending love, support and encouragement, and to my children Layla and Alfie for teaching me so much about myself.

About the Author

Dr Guy Meadows is founder of The Sleep School and is a sleep physiologist with a PhD from Imperial College, London. Having researched and worked in sleep for over twelve years, he has successfully treated over a thousand clients and spent over 12,000 hours working with insomniacs in one-to-one clinics, workshops and retreat environments. Dr Guy has been running The Sleep School for over eight years.

He graduated with a first class BSc Honours degree from Glamorgan University, then an MsC (Distinction) at Kings College London in Human and Applied Physiology before completing his doctorate. Whilst studying at Imperial College, London he worked in the sleep research laboratories of the Royal Brompton and Charing Cross Hospitals where he investigated the effects of sleep on the regulation of the human brain.

Dr Guy Meadows is a resident expert on Channel 4's *Bedtime Live* TV programme and is passionate about helping people to get great sleep.

CONTENTS

What established professionals and medical practitioners say about *The Sleep Book*:

'Dr Guy Meadows teaches a revolutionary new method for combating insomnia. His approach is non-pharmacological and hugely successful. This book will be life-changing for anyone who struggles with their sleep.'
Professor Tanya Byron
Chartered Clinical Pyschologist, author and broadcaster.

'Sleep problems affect 25% of the UK population and lead to 30 million frustrated trips to the GP. This book is a lifeline to anyone who struggles with their sleep. Dr Guy Meadows' radical new approach to curing insomnia is incredibly effective and, even better, it is natural – no pills, potions or props necessary.'
Dr Hilary Jones
General practitioner, Health Editor on ITV's Daybreak *and writer on medical issues.*

'Sleep isn't something you consciously do – you have to be awake to do things consciously. Sleep is something your body does when you move your mind out of the way ... What you have in your hands is a truly new approach. In this spectacularly well-written book you will have a door opened that you may not have realised exists. You will learn *how* to get your mind out of the way ... Put your sleep struggle into the hands of this brilliant clinician, and let's get going. Let's learn how to do nothing.'
Steven C. Hayes, PhD
Co-developer of ACT, Nevada Foundation Professor at the Department of Psychology at the University of Nevada and author of Get Out of Your Mind and Into Your Life.

The Sleep School Testimonials

'Having experienced insomnia for as long as forty years, it has been a delight to enjoy satisfactory sleep employing the techniques learnt whilst attending one of The Sleep Schools workshops. The techniques are subtle but effective. I am convinced that the techniques used will eventually become universally accepted practice amongst medical professionals.'
David (UK)

'I would recommend Dr Guy and The Sleep School to anyone who has wrestled with the insomnia. He's professional and obviously an expert, however his techniques are both easy to understand and if you persevere I believe they will be long-lasting.'
Suzie (Australia)

'The time I spent with you last month was the best money I have invested in a very long time! The mindfulness and acceptance technique you taught me has not only improved the quality and duration of my sleep; it has fundamentally changed the way in which I deal with life. Now when I go to bed, I am a sleep within minutes and whilst I still wake up a couple of times during the night, I fall back to sleep very quickly. Thank you for enriching my life!'
Rachel (UK)

'When I started experiencing insomnia about 2 years ago I thought nobody could help me with getting over it until I contacted The Sleep School. The techniques he taught me helped me understand there was nothing to be afraid of, but most importantly he under-

stood what I was feeling at that point of time when it seemed to be no one could. Nowadays I am enjoying of much better sleep and living my life again.'
Maria (Chile)

'I had been suffering from insomnia on and off for about 3 years, and it had been particularly bad over the last 12 months. My insomnia has gone and I am living a more mindful, relaxed and happier life. I highly recommend Dr Guy if you are suffering from insomnia, to get your life and enjoyment of it back again is amazing. I feel like a normal person again!'
Helena (UK)

'Brilliant! Did not know what to expect when I walked in, but Dr Guy managed to show me a completely new way of understanding and coping with insomnia. This new perspective aided by logical, calm methods has improved my sleeping no end!'
Sam (UK)

'Well the first thing I should say is thank you for your time, effort and energy, you have helped me to get back on track, giving my life purpose and meaning again. I have been sleeping almost every night and am now not going through life sleep deprived. I did have a moment after starting my new job, when my sleep started to take a turn for the worse. But I re-read all my notes and started doing the exercises that you have taught me more regularly again and before I knew it I was back to sleeping. My anxiety has also reduced dramatically and when I feel that I am becoming a little anxious the first thing I do is notice it and because I am no longer afraid of it, it quickly dissipates and I am able to continue on without feeling overwhelmed.'
Henry (Canada)

'When I first went to The Sleep School I was sick and tired of being sick and tired. I was only getting 2 to 3 hours of sleep per night. I now sleep 7 to 8 hours most nights. I haven't had a sick day from work in 6 months. The programme that got my sleep back on track also changed my perspective and meditation has become part of my daily life. I recommend this program to anyone who is suffering from insomnia.'
Jessica (UK)

'Having been an Insomnia sufferer for the majority of my life I really believed that I may have been a lost cause, and so The Sleep School was a last roll of the dice for me. I didn't have very high hopes at the out-set but within the first three weeks I was sleeping better than I had probably ever slept in my life, and it was all down to very practical, simple and achievable techniques. I feel that I have now really regained control over a very major part of my life, and I can't recommend Dr Guy Meadows highly enough.'
Simon (UK)

'I would recommend The Sleep School to anyone who suffers with insomnia – they really can help you get your life back. Thank you Dr Guy you have been my saviour.'
Katharine (UK)

'Firstly to say thank you for your support and help. I have reached a point I didn't think possible with my sleep. I am sleeping better now and although I do have the odd 'bad night' it doesn't impact on me the way it used to. The mindfulness exercises have given me the opportunity to slow down and appreciate the moment, instead of letting my mind race about and create situations in my head that aren't real.'
Aziz (UK)

INTRODUCTION
The Sleep School's Insomnia Cure

*'How do people go to sleep? I'm afraid
I have lost the knack'*

Dorothy Parker

If you ask a good sleeper what they do to get to sleep, chances are they will shrug and say, 'Nothing.' They simply put their head on the pillow; if they wake, they might turn over, have a sip of water or go to the loo, but they just sleep without thinking about it.

If you ask an insomniac what they do to get to sleep, they will give you a long, detailed list of what they do during the day, how they wind down before bed and what they do during the night, and yet they still don't sleep.

It doesn't seem fair, does it? But the truth is, most of the things insomniacs are advised to do to cure their insomnia are never going to work if they do those things alone. That's because the mainstream approach is based solely on doing – focused on how to get rid of your insomnia by changing things in your life. At first this is exactly what you want to hear as an insomniac because you want to be free from the pain and suffering that can come from not sleeping. However, while many of the suggested changes might sound like the right things to do – such as giving up caffeine and alcohol, avoiding late nights, slowly winding down and performing relaxation techniques before bed – in the end they can inadvertently put your insomnia on a pedestal.

Sleep becomes more about doing stuff and less about actually sleeping, which for normal sleepers is effortless. If you have followed lots of insomnia advice yet still found yourself wide awake, then you probably also felt a sense of confusion, failure, frustration or anxiety, all of which doubtless kept you even more awake.

You've probably been told that if you can block out your thoughts, get rid of the anxious feelings and control your pounding heart, you will be more relaxed and therefore more likely to sleep. While these things do make it more difficult to sleep, they're not the problem. Struggling to sleep is.

Think about those times when you have been awake all night struggling to sleep, but then fell to sleep just before the alarm went off. When you ask an insomniac why they slept at that point, they will say that the night was ruined anyway, so there was no point in struggling anymore. While this is incredibly frustrating for you to experience, from the point of view of what causes insomnia it is illuminating.

What I learnt from listening to people like yourself and from my own bout of insomnia is that if the focus of your life becomes getting rid of insomnia, you can paradoxically remain stuck in your insomnia.

Good sleep comes about from doing nothing other than getting into bed and putting your head on the pillow, and the secret to good sleep is to relearn how to do precisely that – nothing.

Armed with the knowledge that good sleepers do nothing, we've developed a five-week programme that can radically improve your sleep. We believe sleep needn't be a struggle.

We'll show you how to stop struggling, face whatever it is that's stopping you sleeping, enjoy good-quality sleep on a regular basis and get back to enjoying your life again.

If you want to sleep well, then you need to start behaving like a normal sleeper. The Sleep School's Five-Week Programme will show you how to:

- Do nothing – stop struggling.
- Let go of trying to sleep.
- Watch and observe your thoughts and feelings without judgement.
- Become more mindful and live in the now.
- Welcome and play with your worries and fears.
- Decide on your new sleeping pattern.
- Stay in your bed at night and enjoy the benefits of resting at night.
- Become a normal sleeper.
- Keep your good sleep on track.

If it's so simple, why do we need a programme to follow? I hear you ask. As I will explain later in the book, we humans are pro-grammed to seek out solutions to our perceived problems, whether on a practical, emotional or mental level. But we can't fix insomnia with this kind of approach. We need to under-stand how the mind works and how the mind sleeps so that instead we can use mental and emotional skills like aware-ness and acceptance rather than creating the perfect sleeping environment or relying on a specific set of relaxation tech-niques. After all, we won't always be sleeping in the same bed or be able to have a lavender-scented bath every night, and yet we'd still like to sleep in those situations. That's the difference with this programme – it's about becoming a normal sleeper once again.

This book is for anyone for whom getting a good night's sleep has become a struggle, whether you find it challenging to fall to sleep, stay asleep or you wake up too early. If your insomnia is caused or associated with a sleep-disturbing medical or psychological condition, this approach can offer you a fresh way of overcoming your sleeplessness. It does not matter whether you have had your insomnia for 4 days or 40 years, following the Sleep School's approach can dramatically im-prove the quality of your sleep.

> The Sleep School's programme is a highly effective, 100 per cent natural approach that will have you sleeping better within 5 weeks.

You'll feel better and more energised simply by taking the first step to understand your insomnia. You'll then see a more marked improvement in your sleep over the remaining weeks of the programme. It is important to remember that this is a gentle process that allows the emergence of natural sleep and trying to force it will only result in pushing sleep further away.

We have helped over a thousand insomniacs to achieve drug-free, good-quality sleep and we can help you too.

'When you're deep in the hole of insomnia, it's hard to see a way out on your own. The Sleep School put my mind at rest and helped me stop thinking about my own insomnia, which was the first step in dealing with the problem. I now have a strategy and mental

exercises to improve how I approach my insomnia.
I still have to deal with bouts of sleeplessness, but that
mental empowerment has helped me more than any
other sleep aid or "traditional" medical approach.'
Mark, Oregon, USA

Revolutionary New Approach

One of the key tools that we use at the Sleep School is acceptance and commitment therapy, or ACT[1]. This is a revolutionary
research-based psychological tool that recognises that it is
our struggle or reaction to pain and suffering that actually
makes them worse. ACT promotes mental flexibility, openness
and curiosity, so rather than struggling against negative
thoughts and feelings, we learn to observe, accept and then
let them go.

The Sleep School has pioneered its use within chronic insomnia because it fits with our realisation that it is the struggle with sleeplessness that worsens insomnia. Traditional
approaches to insomnia, such as cognitive behaviour therapy,
or CBT, unhelpfully focus on trying to get rid of the symptoms
associated with poor sleep. CBT's focus is to block out or challenge your thoughts or remove anxious feelings. When it
comes to the struggle with sleeping, however, the thoughts
and feelings end up coming back stronger, in greater numbers
and with more frequency. Your energy is inadvertently put into
trying to get rid of what you *don't* want, rather than into what
you do want, which is to sleep.

The ACT model accepts that it is perfectly natural for you
to want to get rid of the pain and suffering associated with
not sleeping. No one likes being awake all night and feeling

exhausted all day. However, it suggests that struggling to control and avoid your insomnia actually makes it worse in the long run. If you are hearing the word 'acceptance' and thinking that I want you to give in to your insomnia, then you would be right, but not in the way you think.

Resignation is a negative state that involves being stuck where you are and not doing anything about it, and this is *not* what I am suggesting. Acceptance is a positive act whereby you are purposefully choosing to do nothing because it is the most helpful course of action or way of solving the problem at this moment in time. The Sleep School's Five-Week Programme will help you to achieve this.

Before we get started, I want to share my surprise encounter with insomnia, which arose after working and researching sleep for many years and always being a good sleeper. It was this direct and painful experience of insomnia that led to the Sleep School's revolutionary sleep method.

I was never 100 per cent happy with the traditional methods and sleep tools that I used in the beginning of my sleep consultancy, even though many were developed after significant amounts of research. Quite simply, they did not help all of my clients to sleep as much as I wanted them to or, more importantly, as much as *they* wanted to.

Eager to find new ways in which to tackle insomnia, I decided to experiment on myself and investigate my own sleep patterns. Being a good sleeper, I thought I was the ideal guinea pig, since I effortlessly did the thing that insomniacs wanted to be able to do.

My whole life now revolved around sleep, with my days spent listening to clients' tales of sleeplessness and my nights spent applying my full attention to my sleep. I felt sure that this would provide great insights. Then one night in bed the thought popped into my head 'What if I become an insomniac too?'

For the first time in my life I was sleepless, unable to switch off. I tried to laugh it off, in the hope that it would pass, but instead other unhelpful thoughts popped in, such as 'I'm the guy who helps other people to sleep and now I can't!' With each new thought my muscles tightened, my breathing sped up, my body became restless and any sleepiness that I'd felt earlier slipped away.

So not only was I wide awake but I was also anxious, which made things worse. I tried to remain calm and applied all of the tools that I taught my clients. I breathed deeply, contracted and relaxed my muscles, tried to clear my mind and told myself that everything was going to be okay, but nothing worked.

I fell asleep in the early hours of the morning, but there in my mind waiting for me when I awoke was the fear of insomnia. I spent the day trying to ignore it, keeping myself busy in the hope that it would just disappear. It stayed with me and magnified when I put my head on the pillow that night.

I tried everything from warm baths to hot milk, but as each one failed, my thoughts darkened to 'I'm the sleep expert – I should be able to fix this!' In a short space of time I had been gripped by not only insomnia itself, but also the fear of not sleeping. The effort I was putting in to sleep had not worked and then it hit me: perhaps I was trying too hard.

I rewound to when I slept well to figure out what I was doing. How did I do it? Really I did nothing special at all. The only thing I did to sleep was close my eyes – there were no special wind-down routines, no getting out of bed in the middle of the night, no sleepy food and certainly no medication. I realised that if I was going to sleep normally again, I had to retrain myself to do what good sleepers do and so get back to doing nothing again. A sense of ease spread through my body, as if I had given it permission to stand down from the fight, and soon after my sleep returned to normal.

This experience was hugely enlightening and gave me a fresh way of looking at the problem. I could see why conventional sleep fixes weren't fully effective and dedicated my work to developing a struggle-free approach to overcoming insomnia.

The programme in this book is the culmination of this work and has now helped over a thousand chronic insomniacs achieve good-quality, natural sleep on a regular basis and it can help you too!

Five Weeks to Great Sleep
Week 1: DISCOVER . . . why you need to stop struggling to start sleeping

Sleeping soundly feels great and all of us are capable of a good night's sleep. In this week we will look at the common triggers for and the symptoms of insomnia, and most radically of all, how your attempts to get rid of them could have inadvertently fuelled your insomnia in the long term.

Insomniacs can be incredibly creative: most have tried everything they possibly can to get to sleep and yet got nothing in return. Here we ask you to stop struggling with your insomnia and try the Sleep School's effective approach to curing it.

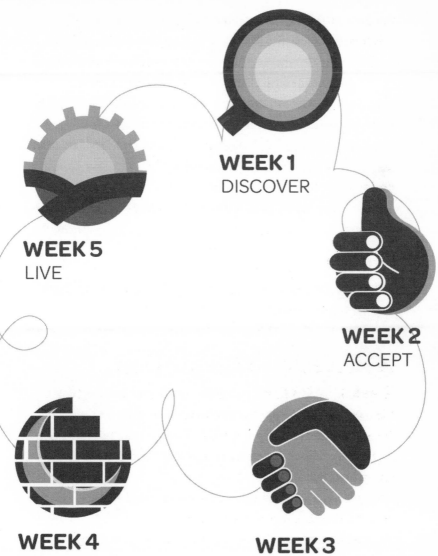

Fig. 0.1 **Five Weeks to Great Sleep**

Week 2: ACCEPT . . . the things you cannot change

Accepting your struggle with insomnia is the most essential step to sleeping naturally. We explain the concepts of control and acceptance, and give you the wisdom to know when to use them helpfully to move you closer to sleep. You will learn the first tool for you to start practising in the day and to use at night if you can't sleep: learning how to live with mindfulness in the present moment, rather than dwelling on the past or worrying about the future. During this week we will train you to be more of an observer, rather than always being so caught up in the whirlwind of your thoughts.

Week 3: WELCOME . . . everything that shows up in your mind and your body

In this week you will learn to meet and greet all of the unhelpful thoughts, emotions, physical sensations and urges that show up in your mind and body when you can't sleep. You will learn to look at your thoughts and choose which ones you follow, rather than buying into them all. Equally you will learn how to make space for the pain and discomfort of not sleeping, rather than unhelpfully struggling against it and amplifying it further.

Week 4: BUILD . . . your new sleeping pattern

Now that you have begun to accept and let go of the struggle you have with insomnia, in this week you will rebuild good sleep patterns. You will determine exactly how much sleep you need and when you need it. You'll start behaving like a normal sleeper again and make constructive and effective changes to your lifestyle.

Week 5 and Beyond: LIVE . . . your days to the full and sleep well every night

This week focuses on living the life you want to live, rather than losing it to an endless battle with poor sleep. You will learn how living your life to the full actually helps you to sleep. To keep yourself on track, you will be given sleep-maintenance tips so you can deal with insomnia if it returns.

How to Use This Book

The Five-Week Programme in this book mimics working on a one-on-one basis at the Sleep School clinic. Each Week will help retrain your brain to achieve natural, deep, refreshing sleep on a regular basis.

The survey below will help you to decide on the strengths and weaknesses of your sleep and which weeks could be most relevant to you. Aim to spend at least one week on each Week to give you enough time to read each section and practise the suggested exercises. Some exercises will suit you better than others and so over the weeks you could practise the tools that most benefit you.

Week 4: BUILD, which you might want to rush to immediately, focuses on rebuilding a normal sleeping pattern but is purposefully left till later in the book to allow you to focus on changing your attitude to and relationship with sleep, before attempting to make changes to your actual sleep.

Reading through all of the five Weeks consecutively has been the most effective way of learning for previous clients. However, if you know that there is a specific Week that you will benefit from most, then you might like to read this first and then return to the others later.

STEP 1 DISCOVER

I struggle to control the quality of my sleep.

I try new things (e.g. pills, potions, rules and rituals) to improve my sleep, but nothing works in the long term.

I don't understand why the things I use to help me to get to sleep don't work.

STEP 2 ACCEPT

I dwell on past poor quality sleep or worry about future sleep and find it hard to switch off my racing mind at night.

I jump from one topic to another and struggle to maintain my focus and concentration in the day.

I realise that I react unhelpfully to try to improve my sleep.

STEP 3 WELCOME

I have negative thoughts about how my poor sleep affects my life and I struggle to get rid of them.

I experience strong emotions (e.g. anxiety) and sensations (e.g. knot in stomach) when trying to sleep or the day after and can't control them.

I find it hard not to give in to unhelpful urges when trying to get to sleep (e.g. watch TV, take a sleeping pill, use alcohol to sleep).

STEP 4 BUILD

I change my sleeping patterns in order to control my sleep (e.g. have a long wind-down, go to bed early or late, lie in or take long naps in the day, sleep alone or get out of bed in the night).

I need my bedroom environment (e.g. light, temperature, noise) to be perfect otherwise I won't sleep.

I change my lifestyle (e.g. changing my diet and not socialising) in order to get myself to sleep.

STEP 5 LIVE

I can't fully get on with life until my insomnia has gone.

I feel that insomnia impacts my daily life negatively (e.g. relationships, energy, work).

I always worry that my insomnia will return and I might have it forever, even when my sleep has improved.

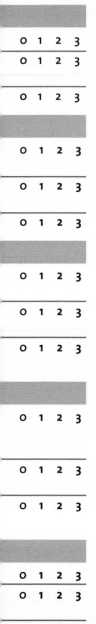

We have suggested a week per step, but really the best plan is to find a pace that works for you and stick with it. If you need to revisit Weeks, then do so, as it will help to consolidate your learning and improve your sleep in the long run.

Each week has its own case study designed to reflect some of the typical problems that you may experience and how to overcome them. These characters have been created using information from the many people who have visited the Sleep School.

Some aspects of this book will be new to you, and some of the suggestions will conflict with what you have previously read or practised, so it will help you to approach every Week with an open mind.

The Sleep School Insomnia Survey

Please read through the statements outlined in the questionnaire and use the following scale to assess your current struggle with sleep and how this book can help you:
0 Never true, **1** Sometimes true, **2** Frequently true, **3** Always true

Results

Add up your score and make a note of it here
....

Your score gives you an indication of your current struggle with your insomnia, so the higher the number, the greater the struggle. Your answers will also identify which of the five Weeks will be most relevant to you. If you have a high number in a particular Week, then you may want to look at that Week more closely.

Keeping a record will help you to track your progress as you work through the book and retest yourself at the end. If you would like to receive your own personalised Sleep School insomnia report please fill out the survey online at www.thesleepschool.org.

DISCOVER
... why you need to stop struggling to start sleeping

'I'm for anything that gets you through the night, be it prayer, tranquillisers or a bottle of Jack Daniel's'

Frank Sinatra

This week we will:

- Learn why the five Weeks are unlike anything that you have ever tried before and how this programme will get your sleep back on track.
- Understand how your insomnia developed and the specific life events or factors that triggered it.
- Examine the mind and body events that commonly arrive when it starts.
- Learn the six common control strategies that unhelpfully aggravate sleep and why what you've tried so far may have made your insomnia worse.

What Is Insomnia?

Insomnia is simply difficulty in sleeping. All of us will experience some form of insomnia in our life, usually only suffering from disturbed sleep for a short time because of a stressful life event. For most of us, sleep returns to normal once the stress has passed. However, for 30 per cent of us, the sleeplessness contines and becomes chronic insomnia.

Chronic Insomnia

Definition: chronic insomnia is defined as difficulty initiating or maintaining sleep, waking early and/or experiencing non-refreshing sleep.

Daytime effects: you might have trouble with concentration, attention and/or productivity levels and/or marked distress such as irritability, anxiety, low mood and general disappointment in your day.

Frequency: insomnia is classed as 'chronic' if it occurs for 3 or more nights per week for a period greater than a month, and typically involves either taking 30 minutes or more to fall to sleep or being awake in the night for the same amount of time.

The most common form of insomnia is known as psycho-physiological insomnia, which means that it is not related to any other mental or physical ill health or environmental cause and involves the interaction between your thoughts, feelings and behaviours (psychology – the mind) and your bodily systems such as those of the heart, lungs, brain and nervous system (physiology – the body). In the past this has been referred to as primary insomnia since it is the primary disorder.

If your sleep disturbance is caused by another mental or physical ill health or environmental cause then it is often referred to as secondary insomnia. This can be seen in people who suffer from mental ill health disorders such as depression or anxiety, which accounts for 40% of insomnia sufferers. Physical ill health disorders such as chronic pain, heart disease or cancer also fall into this category. Insomnia can also occur secondary to environmental disturbances such as chronic noise pollution.

In many instances the treatment of such disorders or resolution of any environmental disturbances can result in a normalization of the sleep, although in some cases the insomnia can outlive the original causal disorder (e.g. the chronic pain, depression or noise is resolved and yet the insomnia remains). If reading this makes you feel that your poor sleep could be associated to another ongoing disorder I urge you to seek medical advice, if you are not already, in addition to reading this book.

How Insomnia Develops

Linda's story, which you can read in the case study given throughout this chapter, is common and shows how easy it is to go from sleeping well to suddenly lying wide awake and confused as to what to do. Having filled in your insomnia survey, you'll already have a good sense of how your own insomnia is for you. Now let's get an understanding of how your insomnia started and, more crucially, why it doesn't seem to be going away. The diagram that follows shows how insomnia starts and develops and is adapted from the Three P Model[2].

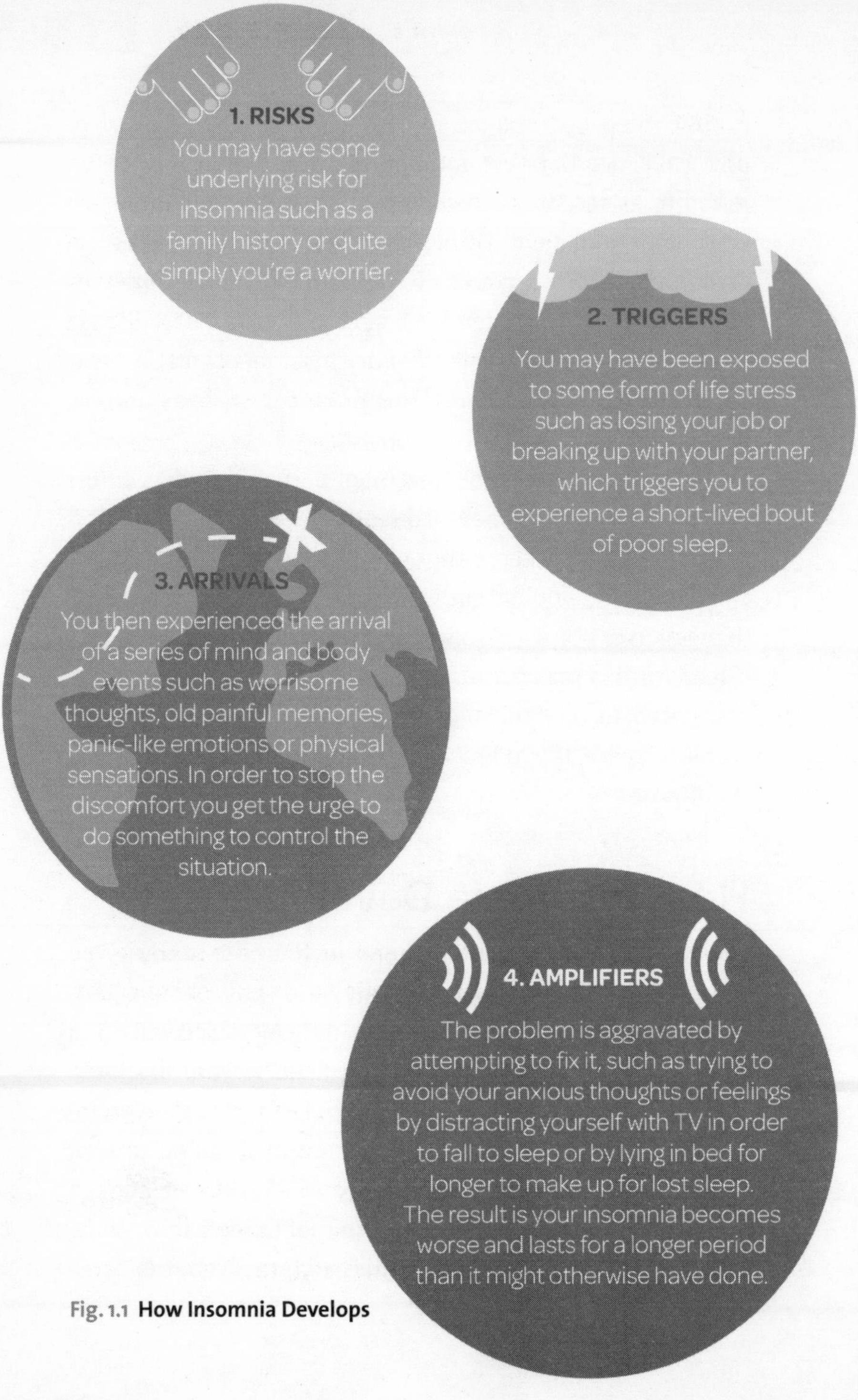

1. RISKS

You may have some underlying risk for insomnia such as a family history or quite simply you're a worrier.

2. TRIGGERS

You may have been exposed to some form of life stress such as losing your job or breaking up with your partner, which triggers you to experience a short-lived bout of poor sleep.

3. ARRIVALS

You then experienced the arrival of a series of mind and body events such as worrisome thoughts, old painful memories, panic-like emotions or physical sensations. In order to stop the discomfort you get the urge to do something to control the situation.

4. AMPLIFIERS

The problem is aggravated by attempting to fix it, such as trying to avoid your anxious thoughts or feelings by distracting yourself with TV in order to fall to sleep or by lying in bed for longer to make up for lost sleep. The result is your insomnia becomes worse and lasts for a longer period than it might otherwise have done.

Fig. 1.1 **How Insomnia Develops**

Risks

The simple truth is that some of us are at more **risk** of developing insomnia than others, in the same way that you might have a risk for heart disease or cancer. Here are some of the things that can increase the likelihood of developing insomnia:

- **Getting older** – as we age, we often experience disorders that disturb sleep such as physical pain or an increased need to use the toilet in the night.
- **Being female** – you're at risk of experiencing potential sleep disturbance from the menstrual cycle, menopause, pregnancy and motherhood. Women also have a greater tendency for worry.
- **Being anxious or a worrier** about everyday life events leads to over-thinking, heightened arousal/wakefulness and sleep disturbance.
- **Being depressed** changes the structure of sleep by reducing (and increasing) the amount required, increasing early awakenings and the amount of dream-based sleep.
- **Family history** – insomnia appears to be hereditary.
- **High arousal level** – people who are 'hyper', 'full of beans' or 'excitable' tend to find it harder to switch off.
- **Genetic predisposition** – anyone who functions best in the early morning (i.e. larks) or the late evening (i.e. owls) and has adapted their life accordingly.
- **Low socio-economic status** – people who have less income, education, occupation and housing opportunities are exposed to a constant level of stress.

Remember, these are risk factors that predispose you to insomnia; they are not a direct cause of insomnia. Just as being overweight does not guarantee that you will suffer from a heart attack, having one or more of the risk factors does not mean you will be an insomniac; they just increase the risk and make you susceptible when a trigger comes along.

Triggers

So we know that some people have a higher risk of insomnia; what happens next is that a stressful life event triggers insomnia.

Any kind of stress can trigger poor sleep. It can be unexpected, such as a stressful day at work, or it can gradually build up, such as planning your wedding. When your thinking mind is overly stimulated, it can create feelings of worry, anger and sadness. They might even cause the release of stress hormones, such as adrenaline, all of which in turn unhelpfully stimulate the waking centre of your brain, preventing you from sleeping.

Take a look at the list of common **triggers** below to see if any of them are familiar to you.

- **Life stress** – anxiety or fear related to relationship problems, work issues, financial worries, pregnancy, childbirth, parenting or bereavement.
- **Medical conditions** – such as angina, cancer, hyperthyroidism, IBS, ME, MS, chronic fatigue, arthritis, back pain or broken limbs.
- **Chemicals** – medication side effects or withdrawal, excessive alcohol or caffeine intake, excess or withdrawal from nicotine or the use of recreational drugs such as cocaine, ecstasy and cannabis.

- **Psychological disorders** – such as generalised anxiety disorder, clinical depression, post-natal depression, post-traumatic stress disorder, obsessive-compulsive disorder, schizophrenia and bipolar disorder.
- **Hormones** – such as menstruation, pre- and post-pregnancy and the menopause.
- **Environmental** – excessive noise, light, temperature or the effect of a change in sleeping environment such as a hotel room.
- **Circadian clock** – any sleep disturbance caused by jet lag or shift work.
- **Other sleep disorders** – in some situations, insomnia can be triggered by another existing sleep disorder, such as snoring, restless legs or bad dreams. To discover if you suffer from another sleep disorder, please refer to the 'Do I have another sleep disorder' questionnaire on our website: www.thesleepschool.org.
- **Childhood** – in some cases insomnia may start due to unknown triggers during childhood.

Thankfully, most stressful situations don't last and sleep patterns return to normal once the stress has passed. When you become an insomniac, what happens is that the period of sleeplessness outlasts the stress. So the initial reason or trigger for why you couldn't sleep is no longer the problem. The real issue therefore is not the trigger, but the subsequent worrying about poor sleep and your reaction towards it.

The good news is that the Sleep School's Five-Week Programme will explain how to respond in the most helpful way towards these worries and get you back to sleeping well.

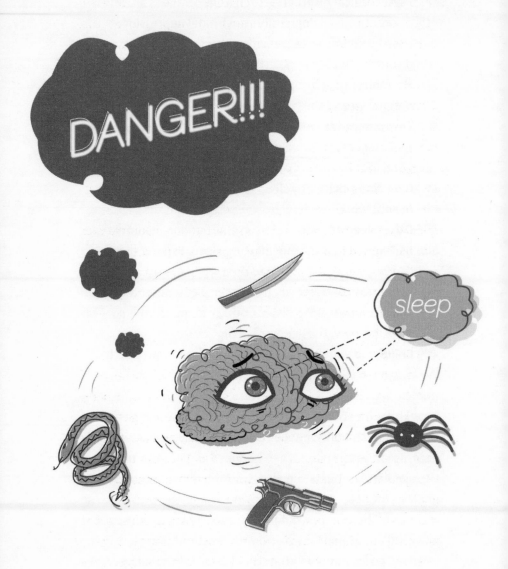

Fig. 1.2 **The Amygdala, our Brain's Prehistoric Threat Detector**

Let's now look at why a stress reaction has such a powerful effect on our sleep and how our brain gets involved too, with the best intentions but with an unhelfpul outcome – insomnia.

Client Case Study: Linda and Her Harmonica

Linda's insomnia was triggered after a stressful day at work left her mind full of worrisome thoughts. She was unable to get to sleep until just before her alarm went off. She had never experienced anything like this before and the next day she felt shattered and anxious that it might happen again. In the back of her mind was the fact that her mother suffered badly from insomnia and she worried that she might be at risk too. Filled with anxiety, she did not sleep again that night and felt wired with adrenaline, her heart pumping so quickly that she thought she was going to have a heart attack.

Arrivals

What happens when we get stressed is that a whole range of unpleasant things turn up or arrive in our mind and body: thoughts, memories, emotions, sensations and urges come crowding in. Not only are they uncomfortable and unwelcome, they also have the capacity to overly stimulate your brain and keep you awake. Lying in bed as your mind races around mulling over your thoughts is not going to help you sleep.

Partly it's our amygdala that's responsible. This is the primitive emotional brain centre responsible for detecting the level of stress and fear in your environment. It releases the stress hormones cortisol and adrenaline, which help us prepare the body to stand and fight or run away in flight, otherwise known as the 'fight-or-flight mechanism'. You will have

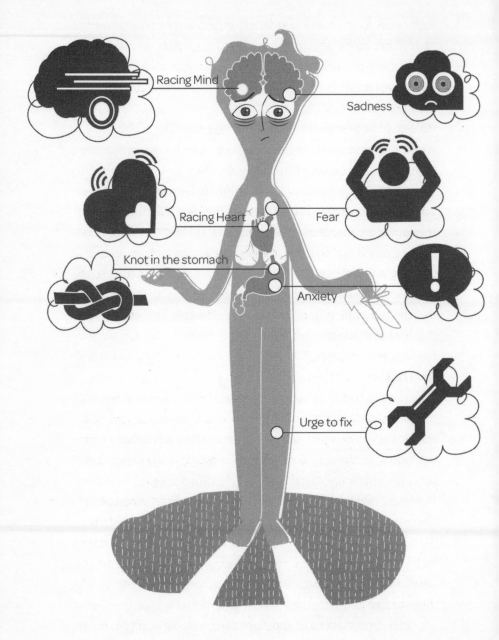

Fig. 1.3 **The Unwanted Arrivals**

experienced it if you've ever been faced with a real emergency. At that moment your mind and body become flooded with new sensations and responses, readying you for action. Your mind speeds up, jumping quickly from thought to thought. Your heart rate quickens to increase the supply of blood, and therefore oxygen and nutrients, to the muscles and brain to assist your escape. Your breathing rate accelerates to increase the supply of oxygen to the body and the removal of carbon dioxide from it. Blood is shunted away from non-essential organs, such as your digestive system, to essential ones, such as your muscles, explaining the knotted stomach feeling. Your palms become sweaty to improve your grip, aiding your ability to climb to safety, and you feel hot as your body attempts to regulate your core body temperaure. Your vision is enhanced by increasing the amount of light received by your pupils.

In this state, you are being 'hyper-aroused', which, as you can imagine, is perfect for fighting off or running away from an attacking predator, but not so good for sleeping!

Once in this state, it is very easy to mistake what we call the **arrivals** – the thoughts, feelings and body sensations that come to you when you can't sleep – as the problem that needs to be dealt with, because everyone knows that you sleep better when your mind is calm and your body relaxed.

We often hear insomniacs say that they would be able to sleep 'if I could just switch off my mind' or 'if I could just stop my heart from pounding' or 'if I could get rid of these anxious feelings' and herein lies the problem. What we tend to do when faced with these unwelcome arrivals is to try to block them or fight them.

Your amygdala can't differentiate between you fighting a lion and you fighting your insomnia and so when your mind regards such arrivals as the enemy and struggles to get rid of them, you go into fight-or-flight mode, which wakes you up more and sends in yet more arrivals! Worse still, if your struggle with sleeplessness continues, you run the risk of such arrivals becoming associated with the act of going to sleep. This means that they show up every night like clockwork because the brain remembers the previous night's struggle and feels it needs to prepare you (by putting you in fight-or-flight mode) for the night ahead.

This also uses up a lot of unnecessary energy, which makes you feel even more tired than if you were simply to lie awake without struggling against it.

SLEEP FACT ☾

The Russian physiologist Ivan Pavlov was the first scientist to identify the concept of respondent conditioning, explaining how your innate emotional and physical reactions to situations can become learnt. His experiments demonstrated how you can take an automatic response such as the act of salivating when you see food and pair it with some other neutral stimulus such as the ringing of a bell.

For example, he showed that if he repeatedly rang a bell shortly before feeding a dog, it quickly learnt to associate the ringing of the bell with being fed and thus would start to produce saliva, irrespective of whether any food arrived. In this situation the bell has become known as a 'conditioned stimulus' because its ringing triggers the now conditioned response of salivation.

Such conditioning explains how both positive and negative responses become learnt. For example, if you get attacked by a dog, you would more than likely feel very scared and reflexly activate your innate fight-or-flight response to help you escape. If you then saw the same dog at a later stage or another dog or even visited the area where it happened, then there is a high chance that you would feel scared again. In this situation, seeing a dog or returning to the same area has become the conditioned stimulus, triggering the unwanted conditioned response of feeling scared.

This conditioning could in part explain why you now experience a fearful response every time you go to bed. In this instance, your 'bell', or conditioned stimulus, has effectively become the act of looking at your watch, entering your bedroom, changing into your bedclothes, putting your head on the pillow or waking up from sleep in the night.

The problem is that this leads to the conditioned response of your amygdala activating your fight-or-flight mode and so pushing you into a state of hyper-arousal or extended wakefulness every time you attempt to fall to sleep or wake up in the night. Naturally such a response is undesirable, which explains why clients go to such lengths to try to get rid of it, as explained in the section that follows.

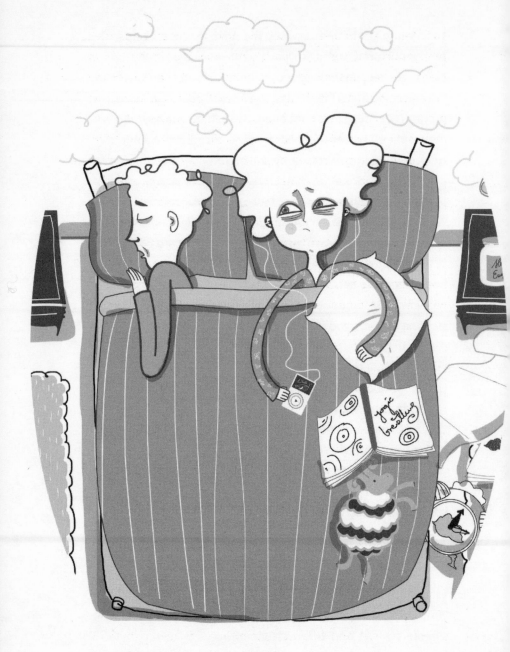

Fig. 1.4 **Pills, Potions, Rules and Rituals**

Case Study Continued . . . Over the next few years Linda tried pretty much every prop, pill, potion, rule and ritual in the hope of fixing her sleeplessness. She tried going to bed earlier, later and even sleeping in during the day. She read all of the guidelines and promptly installed black-out blinds, started wearing earplugs, removed the clock from her bedroom and even bought a new mattress. Her bedtime routine became a military operation, with everything from a warm bath, a milky drink and yoga stretches perfectly timed to get her into bed at the same time every night without fail. She cut out all caffeine, alcohol and sugar from her diet and took up running to tire herself out. She learnt relaxation strategies such as deep breathing and muscle relaxation in the hope of getting herself to sleep. In the end she visited her doctor, who gave her some sleeping pills with the promise of getting her sleep back on track.

Amplifiers

Used in moderation, control strategies can be a helpful way of improving the quality of your sleep. However, if used to excess, they can become the thing that keeps you awake. There are many coping strategies that insomniacs use when desperate to sleep. It is easy to fall into the 'I will do anything to get rid of my insomnia' trap. Coping strategies include using any tool, technique, potion or pill that offers the promise of escape from insomnia, irrespective of how helpful or even harmful they may be.

We call them **amplifiers** because even though they're meant to help, they often don't, and they may even increase your level of wakefulness. Faced with the prospect of another sleepless night and the overwhelming urge to do anything you can to sleep, you may become short-sighted about the

long-term effects of the strategy you have adopted and become unable or unwilling to see any harm you may be doing.
Time to face the facts: your best efforts may be making your
insomnia worse.

The Sleep School has identified six common actions that
can amplify your insomnia:

1   Changing Your Sleeping Patterns

This may include:

- **Spending too long in bed,** as this weakens and
  fragments your sleep.
- **Keeping irregular sleep timing.** Chopping and changing
  your sleep pattern – by going to bed and getting up at
  different times.
- **Napping excessively during the day.** If you nap for less
  than 20 minutes and take a nap no later than 3 p.m., then
  power-napping can be helpful. Beyond this it runs the
  risk of weakening your nocturnal drive to sleep at night.

Sleep patterns are covered in greater detail in Week 4, when
you will build your new sleep pattern.

2   Adopting Unhelpful Habits

This includes any activity to control your sleep that will inadvertently fuel further wakefulness.

Manual activities

These are things that can encourage sleep. For example, reading a book in low light will cause your eyes to become heavy
and increase your desire for sleep. Having a warm bath will

relax your muscles and help to lower your core body temperature. A warm cup of milk or a herbal drink can be comforting and have certain sleep-promoting properties. However, if you are doing these things to get to sleep, you are falling into the controlling trap whereby you become reliant on them.

Electrical activities

Activities such as watching TV, listening to the radio, searching the Web or playing games on your smartphone will keep your brain stimulated and are therefore not conducive to sleep. However, many insomniacs use these as control strategies to help distract their minds from not sleeping. What starts out as an infrequent use of TV to distract a racing mind can soon become a nightly habit that over time loses its effectiveness. Many insomniacs can't sleep unless they have the TV on and end up watching it all night. It is easy to see how your short-term efforts to get some sleep can result in a long-term problem that pushes sleep further away.

Social interaction

We now have the capacity to be connected to the outside world even while lying in bed at night. With a few clicks you can be Tweeting, texting or Skyping with other insomniacs on one of the many insomnia forums. This connection can come as a huge sense of relief and an antidote to the loneliness of the night. However, as with electrical activities, the stimulation involved and the level of brain activity required makes this something you should do during waking hours only, and certainly something that you need to let go of if you are serious about being able to sleep.

Being active

Many insomniacs get up to work, check emails, eat, make a drink, go to the loo, do yoga or other exercises or just wander around the house. Getting out of bed and being active can help to lessen your thoughts or to feel less anxious during a long night without sleep. However, like the other unhelpful coping strategies we've discussed, it is not a long-term solution, and your unwanted thoughts and feelings are simply waiting for you when you return to bed. When this happens, you don't know what to do other than get out of bed again. If this becomes a pattern, then a second problem emerges whereby your brain begins to associate the night-time with getting out of bed and being active rather than resting in bed and sleeping. Learning how to be in bed with your fears and let go of the need to escape the bedroom is therefore key to sleeping well in the long term.

Environmental products

Controlling your sleeping environment is another common strategy. We sleep best in quiet, dark, comfortable surroundings and so it makes sense to set up our bedrooms in this way. Insomniacs often go a step further, using an eye mask or black-out blinds to eliminate light, using earplugs or noise-cancelling machines to block out noise, or constantly buying new pillows and a better mattress to improve their comfort.

It's very easy to begin to use these strategies in an excessive manner and to become reliant on them in order to sleep. It could be argued that needing to use earplugs or an eye mask is not the worst thing in the world, but more often than not they are just one of many props that contribute to the general loss of trust in your own ability to sleep.

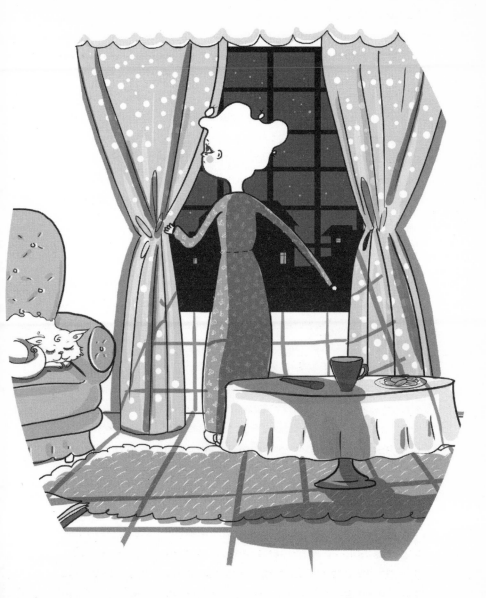

Fig. 1.5 **Avoiding Bed in the Middle of the Night**

The American psychologist Burrhus Frederic Skinner was the first to describe 'operant conditioning', which is the way in which the consequence of your behaviour (i.e. reward or punishment) determines your future behaviour. Examples of this can be seen everywhere in life. For instance, you are more likely to continue working hard if you receive praise than if you don't, or you are more likely to continue with a diet if you lose some weight as a result.

The consequence of your actions therefore affects the way you learn and the way you choose to live your life. Earlier in this week you learnt about Pavlov's respondent conditioning, in which the power of the initial trigger determines your reflexive behaviour in the future, such as constantly feeling scared every time you encounter a dog due to the lesson learnt during the initial attack.

How you behave towards dogs after this event also determines the power and longevity of this response and explains the role of operant conditioning in your learning. For example, if you chose to avoid all dogs in the future, you would have the short-term benefit of not feeling scared but would run the risk of the long-term consequence of always being afraid of dogs. In contrast, if you decided to make contact with dogs again and learnt that not all dogs are harmful, such fears could diminish.

In the same vein the development and maintenance of your insomnia is dependent on the consequences of your actions. For example, if watching TV or taking a sleeping pill helps you to get some sleep in the short term, this desired consequence (i.e. the removal of your unwanted insomnia) reinforces such potentially unhelpful behaviours. This means that you are more likely to use them again and become reliant on them to sleep, something that weakens your trust and pushes natural unaided sleep further away in the long term. At this point it can be seen that the solutions begin to become part of the problem. The challenge comes in being able to look beyond the obvious short-term benefits promised by unhelpful coping strategies and so adopt more workable, longer-term methods.

Mind games

Counting sheep in your mind to induce sleep is one of the most well-known and basic sleep techniques. It works by providing the mind with a monotonous, non-stimulating task to focus on and therefore distract from the worries keeping you awake. Similar techniques include counting backwards from 300 or using your imagination to create an absorbing fantasy.

Such techniques can be reasonably effective for the normal sleeper who easily buys into the distraction and falls to sleep. However, if used excessively, the intention of trying to make yourself sleep and the avoidance of dealing with what shows up in the night will make such techniques unworkable and problematic.

Clock-watching

Clock-watching is a common coping strategy but yet another that aggravates poor sleep. Just as you use the clock in the day to organise your life, monitoring the clock at night can become a way of trying to control your sleep. Many insomniacs use the time as a measure of how good or bad the night is turning out to be and therefore as an indication of whether to deploy further coping strategies.

Many create unhelpful rules such as 'If I have not fallen asleep within an hour, then I will take another pill', or 'If two hours go by, then I will get out of bed', or 'If I have been awake all night, then I will phone in sick and turn off my alarm.' Continuously calculating the time does not help you to fall to sleep and, if anything, can result in greater levels of anxiety and wakefulness.

3   Taking Pills and Potions

Pills and potions include any substance that you use or have become reliant on to control your sleep and therefore have inadvertently made part of the problem. This group includes prescribed and over-the-counter medication as well as alcohol and illegal drugs. I have grouped them together in the 'pills and potions' category because all have the capacity to induce harm to your body if used consistently over a long period of time. In fact, if you look at the unwanted side effects discussed over the following pages, many have the capacity to induce harm in the short term as well. I must stress that if you are currently using any one of these props and thinking about changing them, you should always consult your doctor beforehand.

The goal of control is to find the fastest and easiest route to solving your problems. Any 'magic' pill or potion that promises to put an end to your pain and suffering without having to do much in return is always going to be appealing and difficult to resist in times of desperation. This explains why the vast majority of the insomniacs who visit me have used one or more of these props in order to control their sleep. Not only have the props failed, in most cases they've become part of the problem and can be harmful to your long-term sleep and health, as I will now explain:

- **Loss of trust.** Pills and potions can be initially effective at getting you to sleep. If the process is then repeated, the reliance on that prop can increase to the point where you soon believe that you can't sleep without it. Props are not a long-term workable solution, which is why a key step in this programme is learning how to sleep naturally again.

- **Negative side effects.** Pills and potions typically come with a range of unwanted side effects, such as next-day grogginess, hangovers, memory loss, dizziness and confusion. Such ill effects are often worse than if you had not slept at all and so the costs soon outweigh any benefits. Aside from not wanting to be reliant on such pills and potions, most clients also worry about the impact they are having on their health. Everyone is aware of the long-term health implications of alcohol and smoking cannabis, but because most sleeping medication is only designed for short-term use, very little data exists as to the potential long-term health effects. This is despite the fact that in the real world many insomniacs use such drugs every night and in some cases for many years. Only now are studies beginning to focus on this and preliminary data suggests that long-term use of some of these medications may in some cases be harmful to your long term health.

○ **Effectiveness.** The quality of sleep you get using medication is not the same as natural sleep, with reductions occurring in both deep and REM sleep. This explains why even if you sleep after taking medication, you will wake feeling unrefreshed. At best it will help you to fall off to sleep a little bit quicker or offer a meagre four or five hours of average sleep. However, if used regularly, you may find you only sleep for two or three hours, as the body builds up a tolerance towards the drug. When this happens, most users will then up their dosage or start to combine it with other drugs in order to achieve the same result. Obviously this is not workable and only leads to greater side effects and dependency in the future.

○ **Rebound.** One of the most unwanted side effects of such pills and potions can be the withdrawal once you decide to stop and the potential rebound insomnia. The most common reason insomniacs find it hard to stop taking medication is because when they try to come off, the severity of their insomnia is much worse than ever before.

How to withdraw from medication

As we have seen, when it comes to taking pills and potions to control your sleep, the costs quickly outweigh any possible benefits. If you are currently taking medication to sleep, then you are probably also thinking about coming off it. Over 90 per cent of the people who come to see me are taking some form of prescribed sleeping pill and their reason for attending the clinic is to come off it and get back to sleeping naturally.

Because withdrawing from medication can be a challenging process, it makes sense to be prepared. The first and most important thing to always do is contact your GP and discuss your exit strategy. They will be able to provide you with the best possible plan to withdraw from your medication. Taking a slow approach is generally considered best. As a rule of thumb, doctors advise a quarter reduction in your dose every couple of weeks. This gives the body time to adapt to the reduced level of chemicals in your bloodstream and minimises the chance of unwanted side effects. Taking your tablets for a few more weeks won't hurt, and if they enable you to get a little more sleep, then it is likely to help your ability to learn all of the tools effectively. However, if your sleeping pills do not help or, in fact, make matters worse due to the side effects the following day, then you might decide to come off sooner. Either way it is vital that you speak with your doctor before making any changes to your medication and understand what the effects might be. Note that this gradual withdrawal can be applied to any of the pills and potions discussed earlier.

In my experience the most successful approach is to gradually come off your medication once you have had time to practise all of the tools in the Five-Week Programme and have built your trust in your natural ability to sleep. Doing so can be helpful as it prepares you for the potential discomfort associated with withdrawing and increases your willingness to experience it. Clients who decide simply to go cold turkey at the start are at greater risk of experiencing rebound insomnia, whereby their sleeplessness is worse than before. In this state it can be tough to get through the day, let alone take on board a new set of skills.

4   Engaging in Internal Self-Talk

Internal self-talk includes any inner voice that you use to control your sleep but that inadvertently wakes you up more. You may or may not be aware of such discussions or even arguments going on in your head, but it is something that most of us do.

For some, internal chatter can be a harmless way of providing yourself with a little encouragement and comfort, and for normal sleepers, it often works to induce a state of sleep. However, if the intention behind the chatter is to try to force yourself to sleep, then it can end up backfiring. For example, on finding yourself struggling to drift off to sleep at the start of the night, you might have tried telling yourself, 'Everything will be okay,' or, 'I managed to cope last week, so I can do it again.' All of this is done in the hope of calming yourself down and allowing sleep to arrive. Unfortunately, the fact that you are having to say this in the first place suggests that everything is not okay, and even if you managed to cope last week, there is still a possibility that you might not cope tomorrow. Such positive reframing can therefore unhelpfully attempt to cover up the reality of your situation and set you up for an even greater fall. Many clients liken it to a battle with their own mind that ends up doubling the thoughts in their head and keeping them awake.

Similarly ineffective are strategies such as trying to lull yourself to sleep with statements like 'I am feeling sleepy' or telling your brain that 'I don't care anymore' in the hope that such false acceptance will bring sleep. Again at the bottom of every statement lies the intention of trying to control your sleep, which will end up keeping you awake.

This is especially true if the self-talk ends up focused on yourself for allowing this mess to occur in the first place, such as saying, 'What is wrong with you? Why can't you sleep like everyone else!' Or worse, 'Loser,' or, 'Snap out of it.' Such chastisement simply heightens your arousal levels and further prolongs your wakefulness. If these sound familiar to you, then later in the book you will learn new ways in which to deal with such unhelpful night-time chatter.

5 Practising Forced Relaxation

Forced relaxation includes any relaxation strategy that you use to make yourself more relaxed in the hope of falling to sleep. This makes complete sense because everyone knows that having a relaxed body and mind is vital when attempting to slip off to sleep. Put me in a relaxing yoga class and it's guaranteed I will be the one battling to keep my eyes open or snoring in the corner at the end. If a normal sleeper performs traditional relaxation exercises, more than likely they will feel very relaxed and sleepy. The annoying paradox is that when you are *not* trying to sleep, it comes easily and therefore the problem lies not in the exercises but the intention behind them. For example, if you are performing relaxation exercises to get to sleep, the chances are you will not because the increase in self-awareness means that you narrate your progress (or lack of) in the back of your mind: 'I don't seem to be relaxing' or, 'My heart is beating faster than before' or, 'Why am I still awake? This is not working' and then finally, 'There must be something wrong with me.' The result, of course, is further sleep anxiety.

Ultimately whenever you are trying to achieve anything in life, your brain can't help but want to measure how close you are to your goal. Sadly, when it comes to sleep, the mere act of assessing your progress wakes you up. Most frustrating of all is the 'I think I'm falling to sleep' thought, which then wakes you up!

Remember, it is the unwillingness to experience the arrivals that come in and the struggle with them that keeps us awake rather than the arrivals themselves.

6   Making Life Changes

Life changes include any change to the way you live your life in order to control your sleep. One of the easiest ways in which to control your sleep is to avoid any situation that could possibly make it worse due to excessive stimulation or worry. While limiting your life in this way may seem like a possible solution, it does not solve the problem and, if anything, can make insomnia worse in the long term. Many insomniacs narrow their lives down almost to the point of extinction, only to realise that they still can't sleep. Next we'll look at some of the typical changes I've seen.

Health and personal growth

Top of the list of health changes include cutting out caffeine, doing more exercise or quitting smoking. While all of these activities can have a positive impact on your health, when performed with the intention of improving your sleep, they run the risk of becoming yet another source of sleep anxiety.

- Cutting out caffeine. Caffeine is a stimulant and drinking too much will keep you awake, which is why insomniacs are told to cut it out. While this may make physiological sense, the reality is that if you love your morning coffee or cup of tea, the thought of not being allowed it can bring on just as much anxiety and therefore stimulation as drinking too much caffeine.

- Taking up exercise will certainly help to increase your natural drive to sleep, but if done to get you to sleep, you can end up lying in bed feeling physically exhausted and yet mentally wired, not to mention annoyed because it has not worked.
- Giving up smoking. Cigarettes are bad for your health, and if smoked in the middle of the night to calm you down, they will wake you up more. However, choosing to give up because you are not sleeping can often make things worse, especially since the withdrawal of nicotine stimulates wakefulness.

While all of these health changes can be helpful, cutting everything out in this reactionary way and deciding to live the life of a monk can put your sleep on a pedestal and fuel further wakefulness.

It's very easy to put your life on hold until you get your insomnia fixed. Insomniacs report giving up volunteering, keeping fit or doing their physio exercises either because they want to put all their effort into fixing their insomnia or because they don't have the energy to do anything else. The key is to live a healthy life that allows for personal growth while experiencing but not worsening your insomnia.

Reducing leisure activities

Night-time activities such as going out to dinner with friends or a movie are often avoided for fear that they will be too stimulating. Many insomniacs stop going out because they worry they will spend the whole time clock-watching and worrying and so be unable to enjoy the evening anyway. Most insomniacs will also sacrifice going away on holiday or staying with friends and family as a way of controlling their fear of being in a new sleeping environment or not being able to perfom their normal wind-down routine.

Some people also opt out of hobbies or sports they enjoy in an attempt to avoid experiencing or exacerbating the feelings of tiredness and sickness associated with insomnia. Again, restricting your life in this way is not a long-term solution and often simply fuels your resentment towards your insomnia, keeping you struggling in the vicious cycle.

Relationships

Another area of life to suffer from trying to control sleep is relationships. Some insomniacs sleep apart from their partners as a way of controlling their sleeping environment. While this might help in the short term, it does nothing for your relationship and can increase your fear of bed-sharing.

In addition, an unwillingness to go out and meet friends, do sports or go on holiday can all interfere with your ability to hold relationships with friends or your partner. With insomnia it is easier to become more reclusive, especially as maintaining friendships requires energy, which many do not have. Some are even put off getting into a relationship in the first place because of the fear of having to share a bed or having to be on form. In the past I have had clients who have put off having children because of the worry of not being able to sleep and cope as a parent. Such stories highlight the real cost that insomnia can incur on your life and why it is important to complete this programme as best you can.

Work and education

With insomnia, work stress or the worry of not being able to perform at work is common. Many insomniacs attempt to control it by choosing to avoid it. This can mean phoning in sick after a poor night, which can then result in a deep sleep because the pressure has been lifted. For others, the fear that their insomnia will worsen if they experience more stress has driven them to turn down promotions at work or to not enrol on a degree course or sit exams. The sad thing is that the fear of not sleeping can literally determine the life you end up living and keep you away from what is truly important to you in life.

Many insomniacs inadvertently allow their poor sleep to dictate the type of work that they pursue. They choose jobs that have flexi-time or become self-employed as it allows them to choose their own working hours and so avoid morning meetings. While such control can avoid unwanted stress, hopefully you can see that it is not fixing the problem in the long term, but merely finding ways to avoid it.

Exercise: What are your amplifiers?

Jot down any of the amplifying actions that you currently use to help yourself sleep. This includes anything from earplugs and eye masks, to alcohol and prescribed medication, or any way in which you limit your life to control your insomnia. Note also any reliance on such props and, as you work through the book, gently begin to let go of them and regain your trust in your natural ability to sleep once more.

Case Study Continued... Linda's desperation to sleep meant that she was ready to try almost anything and as a result was blind to the obvious amplifying effect of trying too hard! This was until one night when she randomly slept for eight hours and could only put it down to playing the harmonica at a friend's house the night before. The next morning she promptly bought a harmonica and booked a set of lessons, but unsurprisingly her poor sleep returned the next night. Thankfully it was at this point that she realised she had gone too far and needed to seek professional help!

Why We Control

By now you have hopefully realised that it is the adoption of amplifying behaviour that keeps you stuck in the vicious cycle of insomnia. As with all the techniques or lifestyle changes detailed above, your main concern becomes whether they work or not. If they do work, even if it's only a couple of hours of extra sleep, such behaviours can get logged by your brain as a possible insomnia cure. You can end up becoming attached to them, believing that you can't sleep without them or, worse still, becoming chemically hooked on them, if using pills to sleep. This is the start of your brain's perception of sleep as a problem to be solved rather than something natural and safe. You can see how easy it is to get trapped in a vicious cycle.

Behaving in a way that makes your insomnia worse seems daft, but in reality you are doing what comes naturally. The evolutionary success of humans is founded on the basic principle that the more control you had over your environment, the greater your chance of surviving. As long as you could

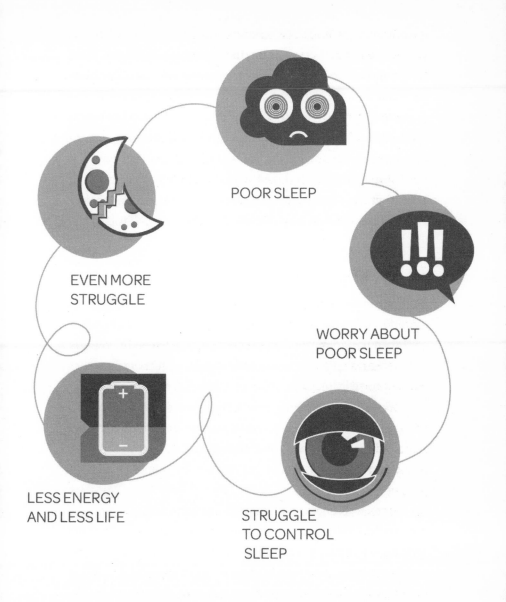

Fig. 1.6 The Vicious Cycle of Insomnia

make a shelter, find food to eat, successfully reproduce and defend yourself, then your life expectancy was higher. To do this, your brain evolved to be able to use every life experience you have as a reference library to solve your problems in the present or future. This meant that when it came to building a shelter, your brain could now rapidly identify the best materials and tools for the job. Amazingly, it could do this even if it had little or no previous knowledge of building a shelter. Being able to process all of this information and organise it rapidly in such a functional way propelled humans to the top of the food chain.

In modern times our basic needs are mostly met, but this has not stopped our brain's ability to constantly predict and problem-solve in all areas of our life, including the quality of sleep. For example, if you feel that you have an uncomfortable bed, then you might decide to buy a new mattress. If you find yourself staying in a noisy hotel room, you might choose to block out the noise by using earplugs or ask to be moved to a quieter room. So you can see how easy it is for your brain to come up with solutions and make changes when you don't like something. As it is so effective, we also exercise this control in our internal world, such as managing unwanted thoughts, feelings and even sleeplessness.

For example, if you get home from work and feel angry or stressed, it can be helpful to distract yourself by doing some exercise or watching a movie. More than likely afterwards you will feel calmer and in a better state to get to sleep. And if you go to bed feeling stressed, then counting sheep or thinking about a past holiday can be a harmless way of distracting your mind and therefore allowing sleep to arrive. Used in moderation, control strategies do 'work', in as much as they can lessen racing minds or calm angry feelings and even help you to fall to sleep.

Ultimately, however, you cannot get rid of stress just by pushing it away or ignoring it, and in fact doing so can often make the problem worse. The reason for this is because the same part of the brain that helps you to build a shelter can also help you to build a chronic sleep problem. When faced with sleeplessness, your brain will rapidly identify the best materials and tools for fixing the job (e.g. 'What pills, potions, rituals and routines can I use to fix this?'). It will compare your current sleep to how it was in the past or project forward to how it may be in the future (e.g. 'If my sleep gets any worse, then I won't be able to cope!'). It will also try to estimate some form of timeline to your actions (e.g. 'If I am not asleep by one o'clock, then I will take another pill').

Your brain is incredibly adept at seeking solutions to your insomnia; however, such a hive of activity is the complete antithesis of sleep. It could be said that your brain's attempts to get you to sleep are literally keeping you awake! The good news is that you are about to learn a new healthier and control-free approach to achieving natural, deep, refreshing sleep on a regular basis.

Case Study Continued . . . One thing for sure was that Linda couldn't be accused of not putting in enough effort, energy, determination or even money to try and fix her insomnia, and herein lay the problem. In her effort to try and control her sleeplessness, the more out of control she became and the worse she slept. The act of going to sleep now involved an elaborate array of pills, props, rules and rituals, which for the most part did not even work, but she was at a loss as to what else to do. By the time she came to the Sleep School, she was reliant on sleeping pills despite the fact that they offered her only a few hours of poor-quality sleep. Plus for her to even consider sleeping, she needed to perform a lengthy wind-down routine to get her in the mood and the room had to be pitch dark, silent and the perfect temperature!

After filling out the Sleep School Insomnia Survey, it became clear to her that rather than helping, her actions had inadvertently placed sleep on a pedestal far out of her reach. Her brain had got used to the constant struggle with sleep and, worse still, now feared it and did all it could to keep her awake. Linda expressed anger at herself for having let the situation get so out of hand, but also felt relief that she no longer needed to continue struggling with her sleep and could start to let go of the unhelpful props that she had acquired. Within a month she felt like a normal sleeper, no longer reliant on pills or props to sleep. Best of all, she now trusted her body to sleep and so it did.

Exercise: Getting to Know Your Insomnia

One of the largest obstacles between you and sleeping well is how you view your insomnia, which determines how you feel and react when you experience it. If you can stop fighting your insomnia, you can direct your energy into allowing natural sleep to emerge and get back to living your life.

For many insomniacs, sleeplessness is the worst thing in the world and something that they would not wish on their enemies. Many describe it with a sense of hatred and loathing, and tell dark stories of how it has ruined their lives. Have a think about what insomnia means to you at this moment in time and then write out your thoughts. How does it affect you and your life right now?

It will be interesting to reread this when you've been through the five weeks of the programme.

When the Solution Becomes the Problem

Often it takes just one poor night of sleep for the seed of doubt to be sown in your mind about your ability to sleep. From here your brain has the capability to predict, problem-solve and panic its way into a state of chronic insomnia. Think back to before you became an insomniac; you probably never even thought about sleep and now you can't stop.

As we've seen over the course of this chapter, problems arise when you start to behave in a way that amplifies your insomnia. Your actions may help to get rid of unwanted thoughts, sensations and urges, and even sleeplessness in the short term, but they end up make sleeping less likely. For example, sleeping during the day may help you to catch up on sleep and feel better, but if continued can eventually get in the way of living a normal life, such as working a nine-to-five job. Equally, having a strict and lengthy wind-down routine may help you to become relaxed and fall to sleep quickly, but it also limits your ability to be with friends or family.

Another problem with such control strategies is that they often don't last in the long term. For example, you might choose to distract yourself from unwanted thoughts in the night by listening to the radio. If you continue to do this every night, you can end up needing to listen to it for longer and longer to achieve the same result. After a while, it can stop working altogether, but you daren't let go of it because of the fear of losing control. The problem is that when one technique fails, your brain has already replaced it with ten others and out of desperation you lie in bed trying them all.

Sleep is a natural physiological process that requires no conscious effort or energy for it to occur, just like breathing or the beating of your heart. Attempting to excessively control your sleep is likened to struggling with quicksand: it costs you a lot of energy and makes everything worse.

The Cost of Your Insomnia

Take a moment now to think about how much effort you have put into trying to control your insomnia and the overall cost to your life so far. If you are anything like Linda, the costs are probably quite high and varied, as seen with the examples below:

- **Emotional** – the rollercoaster of emotions, moods and feelings that you experience when continually struggling to improve your sleep.
- **Energy** – the energy needed to constantly battle against your poor sleep and the extra effort required to be able to live a so-called 'normal' life.
- **Life** – the loss of living in the process of trying to control your sleep.
- **Health** – the impact that not sleeping and struggling with sleep has on your health.

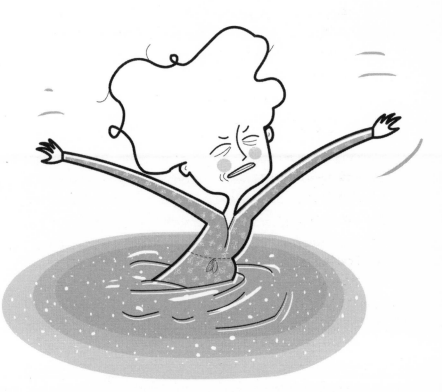

- **Financial** – the financial cost of every device, technique, book, therapy or substance that you have purchased to improve your sleep.

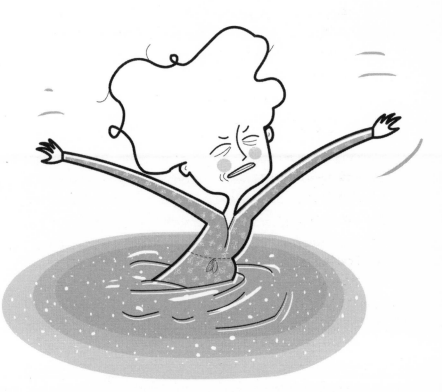

Fig 1.7 **The Insomnia Struggle**

The Way Forward

Hopefully you are beginning to realise just how little control you have over your sleep. Realising the high price of your endless struggles to control your insomnia and discovering that such actions could have even played a part in its development, you may experience a wave of yet more unwanted arrivals, such as despair, self-pity, depression, helplessness, hopelessness, anger or just a sense of numbness. This is a perfectly natural response; just respect the feelings that you have and don't waste any further energy trying to get rid of them. It's time for you to get out of the vicious cycle!

You can't change your insomnia risk factors, such as being born into a family with a history of sleeplessness. Nor can you change the past events that triggered it to occur. Equally you can't predict the thoughts and emotions that will arrive in your head, let alone control them. The only thing you can control is how you behave, and the key is to make sure it is helpful. How you act towards your insomnia will determine your insomnia, and it is your actions that will release you from the vicious cycle and put you on the right track towards deep sleep.

As you work through this book, you will learn longer-term coping strategies for overcoming your insomnia that will help you develop a strong and robust sleeping pattern. It's time to move on to Week 2: ACCEPT to discover a way to improve your sleep, enabling you to use your valuable energy for living your life.

ACCEPT
...the things you cannot change

'A poor life this, if full of care, we have no time to stand and stare'

William Henry Davies

This week we will:

- Show that the key to great sleep is to stop struggling and do nothing.
- Understand the barriers that stand in the way of great sleep.
- Learn how to use mindfulness tools in the daytime and the night so that you respond in a more helpful way when you can't sleep.

Losing Control and Finding Sleep

So we now know that we can't control our sleep and that in many instances trying to do so only makes it worse. Understanding this fact does not stop you from continuing to try to control your sleep; after all, it is what you have evolved to do, and applying control is proven to work in so many other life situations.

The fact is, it does not work for insomnia and so another way is needed if you are to escape its vicious cycle. Acceptance means that you choose not to struggle with your poor sleep and all of the pain and suffering that come with it.

How does this help you sleep? In the short term it means you stop the physical tossing and turning, emotional fretting, over-thinking or excessive energy expenditure, all of which keep your brain awake and prevent your entry into peaceful slumber. In the long term it re-associates the act of going to bed with sleeping soundly, so that you fall to sleep soon after your head hits the pillow and stay asleep with little disturbance until you wake in the morning. The additional benefit is that by not struggling, you save energy for the day ahead, which you can then choose to put back into living a rich and meaningful life, something that has a calming effect on your brain, increasing the likelihood of more restful sleep the next night. You sleep better on a bed of ease!

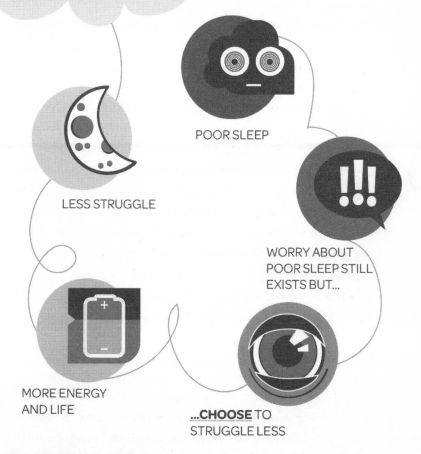

THE ARRIVAL OF GREAT
SLEEP, MORE ENERGY,
AND A RICH &
MEANINGFUL LIFE

POOR SLEEP

LESS STRUGGLE

WORRY ABOUT
POOR SLEEP STILL
EXISTS BUT...

MORE ENERGY
AND LIFE

...**CHOOSE** TO
STRUGGLE LESS

Fig. 2.1 **Breaking the Vicious Cycle**

Client Case Study: Carlos and His Unwillingness

When he came to see me at the Sleep School, Carlos was desperate to find a solution to his poor sleep, which had been plaguing him for just under a year. Like most insomniacs, he would do virtually anything to get a good night's sleep and was ready to fight his insomnia. I explained to him that rather than fighting it, I wanted him to accept it, as it was his continued struggle with it that had been keeping it strong. This came as a real shock, especially the part where I told him that I needed him to have some sleepless nights so that he could get to know his insomnia 'demons'. He left feeling very deflated and disheartened because he had thought I was going to give him some weapons with which to fight.

That night he used a few of the tools that I had given him, only to have his worst fears confirmed when they 'did not work' because they did not stop the arrival of his anxiety and other unwanted guests. The next day he called me to explain how he had been awake all night and how accepting his anxiety had made it feel stronger than it had been in a long time. He said that while he imagined my techniques worked for some people, he was not ready to accept his insomnia and that he would pursue other approaches.

So What Stands Between You and Sleeping Well?

So now we are at the point in the programme where you hopefully understand how your actions can amplify sleeplessness and that accepting your insomnia is half the battle to curing it. The question is, will you continue to behave in the same way, or are you willing to change?

The good news is that the main thing sitting in your way is *you* and you have the power to change it! Here are some of the things you might be feeling right now – they're pretty common and must be overcome to move you past being stuck in insomnia:

○ **I will fail.** Fear of failure is one of the biggest reasons for struggling with sleeplessness. This can either be because you fear you will fail to cope the next day and the potential consequences of that, or you fear simply not being able to perform the act of sleeping like everyone else. The Sleep School's Five-Week Programme paradoxically teaches you to be willing to fail at sleeping because it is only when you can accept wakefulness that you can sleep.

○ **It will hurt.** It goes without saying that if you don't sleep, then you don't feel particularly good the next day. Excessive tiredness, aches and pains, and mood swings are all very common. In reality though, while uncomfortable, most sensations experienced through sleeplessness do not cause actual physical hurt, despite your mind telling you otherwise. Let go and be open to experiencing such discomfort rather than wasting your energy struggling with it.

○ **I can't sleep without pills or props.** Loss of trust in your own natural ability to sleep due to a reliance on medication can be a huge barrier for many poor sleepers, especially if learning to sleep naturally involves experiencing withdrawal symptoms and worse sleep in the short term. If this is the case for you, then you will soon be learning tools to let go of your reliance and start sleeping soundly. As we saw in the previous chapter, it is really important to get help from your GP at the same time as doing this programme.

- **I'm a lost cause.** Complete doubt in one's ability to sleep normally again is very common. Countless failed attempts to resolve the problem and ensuing poor sleep can chip away at even the most optimistic of individuals. Being resigned to your insomnia will keep you stuck in this state. Accept your insomnia if you want to move on.

- **My mind is too strong.** Often people blame their own minds for being too strong-willed to overcome their insomnia. If this is the case for you, then it is important to remember that it is your own mind that is telling you this and therefore it is your choice as to whether you believe it or not.

- **Why me?** In the middle of the night it is easy to believe that you are the only one who can't sleep and that you have in some way been singled out for torture. The reality is that you are not alone, with up to 30 per cent of the population also suffering. Once again it is your choice as to whether you buy into this thought or start to let it go.

- **It's not the right time.** Many clients will delay their own progress because it is not the right time (e.g. they have a lot of stress on at work, have a new baby or are going on holiday). If you are honest with yourself, there will never be a 'perfect' time to start a programme of change, and delaying is often just another form of avoidance.

○ **I'm too tired.** Tiredness can be a real barrier to your progress because it can lower motivation and your willingness to experience discomfort. For example, the extra tiredness commonly experienced in the first few sleepless days after coming off pills can be enough to drive people to give up and revert back to tolerating a few hours of drug-induced sleep and next-day grogginess instead. Being unwilling to experience short-term tiredness means that you will never know what it feels like to be fully refreshed in the long term.

Experiencing such barriers could be likened to running a marathon or any distance whereby you begin to feel challenged beyond your natural comfort zone. At the start you probably feel in good spirits and full of energy to get to the finish line. However, after a while your legs begin to ache, you start to get cramp, you get out of breath, and you are sweating profusely. Suddenly the task in hand is much more uncomfortable than you expected and your mind creates barriers blocking your way. At this moment you are faced with a choice of whether to stop running or keep going. If you choose to carry on, it is not because you like pain and discomfort or you want more of it, but rather you see it as an inevitable part of the journey. You decided to run this race and so you are willing to own the discomfort that comes with it.

In the same vein, as you work through this programme, and even as you lie awake choosing not to rely on your usual armoury of props and pills, you may experience the same old worrisome thoughts about the next day, or the familiar pang of anxiety in your stomach, or the urge to escape by going downstairs and watching TV. At that moment in time you are faced with a choice of whether to give in to your old props or continue on your new path. If you decide to continue, it is obviously not because you enjoy the discomfort, but because you choose to act in the most helpful way to becoming a great sleeper and living a more satisfying life in the long term.

'I feel as though I've been given my life back. I no longer dread going to bed anymore, and there may be nights when I don't sleep so good, but rather than fight them, this programme has shown me how to accept them and at least get some rest.'
Karen, London

Original or Amplified Pain

While the benefits of acceptance and facing our fears are clear, many of us still struggle with the idea of letting go of control, even though it is something that we do in our everyday lives. You probably already accept a level of discomfort as a way of solving problems and moving forward. For example, you may have gone on a diet in order to lose weight and therefore been open to experiencing the sensations of hunger or the craving to eat junk food without actually acting upon them. You may choose to go to the gym or do exercise to get fit and therefore be willing to endure the physical pain that comes with it. Perhaps you've been willing to accept the symptoms of withdrawal from nicotine for the sake of giving up smoking. If you have ever been in a relationship that has broken up you will know how important it is to accept the pain of the break up before you can move on and find a new partner. The same goes for losing your job, only by being open to experiencing the hardship that often comes with it can you find it in yourself to start looking again. Finally, I am sure that some of you will have even experienced the death of a loved one and noticed that it was only when you allowed yourself to really feel the pain of grief that you were able to start living your life again.

Accepting insomnia requires being willing to sit with, lean into, make space or open up to the pain and suffering that you have been trying so desperately to control and avoid. By doing so, you'll allow yourself to sleep naturally and move forward with your life.

In this situation it can be helpful to try an ACT (acceptance and commitment therapy) view of your pain and suffering as either 'original' or 'amplified'. Original pain refers to that which naturally shows up because of your insomnia risks, triggers and arrivals. In contrast, amplified pain refers to the additional pain and suffering that shows up every time you unhelpfully attempt to control and avoid your original pain, as we explored in the previous Week.

For example, you can't change the fact that you are an anxious person and that this puts you at a slightly greater risk of insomnia than others. Neither can you turn back the clock so that you never had that argument with your partner that caused you to be awake worrying, triggering your insomnia to start. You also can't stop the fact that for the time being your brain associates the night-time with wakefulness because this is what it has learnt to do. You can't stop the arrival of thoughts such as 'If I don't sleep, I won't be able to cope tomorrow' or 'I am going to die if I do not sleep soon.' You can't stop the feelings of loneliness and anger in the night, and depression and desperation during the day. You can't stop the physical knot in your stomach that arrives at the thought of not sleeping. You can't stop the urge to take a pill in the hope of sleeping a few hours or having to deal with life feeling excessively tired. Finally, you can't change the wider impact that not sleeping has already had on your life, such as your inability to hold a relationship, do your job and even maintain your health.

This is a pretty heavy list describing things that I am sure you'd not wish on even your worst enemy. It's crucial that the discomfort that exists with regard to your insomnia needs to be accepted before you can start to move on. As the American psychologist Carl Rogers said, 'When I can accept myself just as I am, then I can change.' Acceptance of the past and the present situation (i.e. the original pain) is the first hurdle to moving your life forward.

The good news is that *you* control the level of amplified pain that you experience because it is nothing more than the product of your unwillingness to experience your original pain. In fact, the majority of your sleeplessness comes from your continued struggle with and attempts to avoid poor sleep, rather than from the poor sleep itself. For example, when you suffer from insomnia it is perfectly normal to experience thoughts like 'If I don't sleep, I won't be able to cope tomorrow.' However, it is your struggle to block the thought from your mind or change it into something more positive that keeps you awake and not the thought itself.

Take a moment to think about your pain and discomfort and how much is original and how much is amplified. For many insomniacs, as much as half the pain they experience is the direct result of their struggle with the original pain.

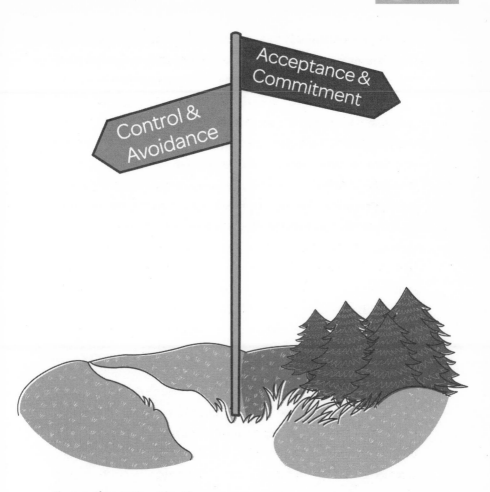

Fig. 2.2 **Choose Your Direction**

You have arrived at a fork in the road and it is time to make a decision on how you plan to act towards your insomnia! You can continue to try to control and avoid your insomnia and continue to amplify your sleeplessness and the impact that it is having on your life, or you can choose to own the original pain and allow natural, deep, refreshing sleep to emerge, along with a new life full of vitality and energy.

Case Study Continued . . . Six months later I received a phone call from Carlos telling me that he was ready to use my approach. He described how during that time he had tried countless things to get rid of his insomnia, all of which promised to fix his sleep and yet didn't. In spite of the wasted time, money and energy, he was very pleased to have been on his journey, as it had allowed him to come to terms with the fact that there are no quick fixes or magic pills. Most importantly, he now accepted that recovering from his insomnia would require him to be willing to face up to the discomfort of not sleeping, which he had been so desperately trying to avoid. He also recognised how accepting this discomfort would probably pale into insignificance when compared with the alternative of continuing to fight his insomnia for the rest of his life.

Isn't 'Acceptance' Just Another Word for 'Giving In'?

For many people, the word 'acceptance' is commonly confused with the more negative state of being resigned. You are resigned to your insomnia if you think that you will never sleep properly again or that you have tried everything and nothing works for you, that your brain has forgotten how to sleep and as a result you are going to stick to sleeping pills and not try anything else.

In this state you are unwilling to help yourself to move forward and only two things can happen: you remain stuck where you are or it gets even worse.

By contrast, acceptance means that you accept that you have insomnia and acknowledge that is simply how things are at the moment. This is far from being resigned or displaying weakness. In fact it is a sign of real strength, since being willing to sit with the original pain that arises in the middle of the night takes a lot of courage. It is often far easier to have another glass of wine, take another pill or watch TV all night and avoid dealing with insomnia than it is to actually choose to stay with it. Deep down, though, we know that while these things might provide a quick fix for the night, they are not a long-term solution.

Like my client Carlos, there will come a time when you will need to face your fears, and while this can be scary and uncomfortable, it can bring a huge sense of relief. On realising that they can stop struggling, insomniacs often describe feeling lighter and more able to float with their problems, rather than being pulled under by them. Being willing to accept your insomnia is therefore not a sign of weakness or some sort of masochistic act, but a justified helpful response to months or years of struggle, wasted energy and missed opportunites in your life.

Making the Most Helpful Response

Your aim is to achieve natural, good-quality sleep on a regular basis. The Five-Week Programme will help you to achieve this by assisting you to make the most helpful decisions for your sleep, meaning ones that move you towards sleepiness rather than away. To do this, you need to be able to carefully choose between your natural evolved tendency for control and the gentle process of acceptance. The Serenity Prayer most eloquently describes this choice:

> *Grant me the serenity to accept the things I cannot*
>   *change,*
> *the courage to change the things I can,*
> *and the wisdom to know the difference.*

Since most of us are quite adept at changing things in our lives that we don't like, the Five-Week Programme is mostly focused on accepting the things we can't change. If you are still unsure, then consider it this way. Imagine you have a noisy neighbour who is keeping you awake with their music. In this scenario there is something for you to control because you can go round to their house and ask them to turn down the music. However, if the noise is coming from your own head because your mind is racing with thoughts, trying to tell your mind to be quiet will often only make your thoughts shout louder. In this situation learning to change your relationship with your thoughts rather than struggling to change them is a more helpful solution.

'Even if I experience wakefulness now, I still seem to be fine the next day, compared to before I started the programme. Before, I would struggle with wakefulness all night and feel exhausted the next day. The thing I have learnt from this is that it's the struggle with wakefulness that really hurts, not the wakefulness itself.'
Richard, London

Hundreds of people have benefited from this programme and are now enjoying good-quality sleep on a regular basis. *You* can too by following the practical tools outlined in the next section.

Mindfulness and Sleep

The tools you are about to learn are a revolutionary way of overcoming insomnia. They are unique in the fact that they are *not* designed to get you to sleep. How they will help you will become apparent as you practise, which you will be encouraged to do during the day and the night.

The first step to accepting your insomnia is to be able to notice yourself struggling in the first place. What you don't see you can't begin to let go of. This may sound obvious, but it is all too easy to fall into a pattern of mindless thinking, where we are completely unaware of things going on around us or our own behaviour.

Often we can be doing something or having a conversation, but our mind is elsewhere. Therefore we have no recollection of the actual task or, worse still, what the other person said! A common one for me is locking the door to my house and walking away and then questioning whether I locked it or not.

At a basic level such mindlessness is relatively harmless and is what happens when you daydream. However, during times of stress, such as when you can't sleep, a lack of awareness of what is going on in the moment can keep you struggling when you don't even know you're doing it. You can spend your day either locked in worry about how little sleep you've had or imagining how bad tomorrow will be if you don't sleep. Night after night is spent trying to work out how to fix your insomnia, and of course this over-thinking literally keeps you awake. Is this how it is for you?

The good news is that you already possess all of the tools you need to be able to see yourself pulling on the rope and then choose to let go. So what is mindfulness? If you gave my daughter a raisin when she was a year old, she would playfully and curiously explore every part of it. Before it got to her mouth, it would have probably visited the inside of her ear or been up her nose. It would have been squished between her fingers or just gazed at for what would seem like an eternity to her impatient parents, who were encouraging her to eat. Living in the moment like this is a slow process of exploration that is outside of normal time. It is free from judgement and is called the 'beginner's mind'. For my daughter, this meant exploring every last detail of her raisin in that moment, rather than thinking about how it compared to past ones she'd eaten or imagining what the next one might be like. She was living in the *now*, and *you* can too!

Unfortunately, as you age, you develop a library of experience against which things can be compared or judged. Your surroundings become more familiar and your life speeds up, resulting in you spending less time in the present moment. You race around under the illusion that if you can do just a little bit more, then you'll be able to rest. As I am sure you already know, such thinking is a trap that results in you going faster and faster. In this state it can be said that you have 'no time to stop and smell the roses' and it is easy to become trapped in your own mind and stuck on automatic pilot.

SLEEP FACT

You don't need to be a Buddhist in order to benefit from mindfulness; it has been used by nearly all world cultures and religions throughout the ages. You just need to be willing to pay attention on purpose to the present moment as it unfolds.

Mindfulness is now taught all over the world, and in recent years a plethora of research has been conducted

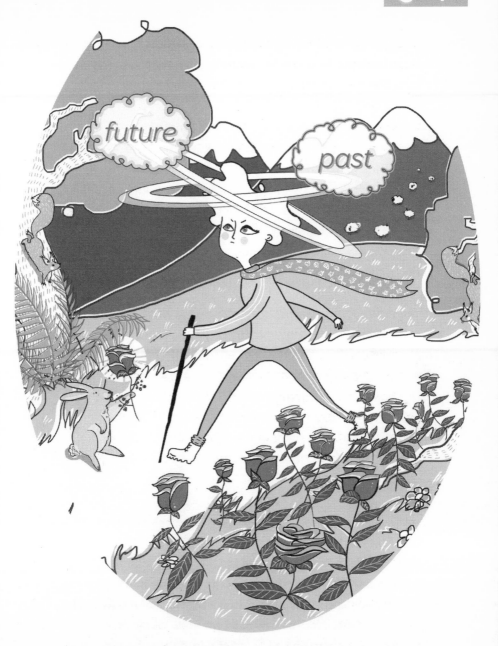

Fig. 2.3 No Time to Smell the Roses

to show its effectiveness at treating a variety of mental and physical conditions, including obsessive-compulsive disorder, chronic pain, anxiety, depression, drug addiction and insomnia.

Like insomnia, many of these conditions are amplified by our unhelpful attempts to control the pain of the here and now, and to find a solution. Mindfulness therefore offers a gentle way of experiencing, owning and honouring such discomfort, rather than struggling to avoid or change it.

Mindfulness is an important element of ACT and is an essential tool in the Five-Week Programme.

'I use mindfulness practices most days now. Apart from my sleep, which is now better than it's ever been, I've found mindfulness practices – e.g. focusing on my breath and noticing my senses – especially useful in the busyness of having two little children. It would be easy to feel frazzled or to over-think, but these techniques regularly help me to come back to the present and help me to stop and enjoy the moments which pass by all too fast!'
Nikki, London

Case Study Continued . . . To help Carlos let go of struggling with his insomnia, he first needed to be able to catch himself in the act. For this I introduced the concept of being mindful of the present moment, rather than always worrying about how bad he slept the night before or how bad tomorrow would be if he had another poor night. He had heard of mindfulness before, but always thought that he would be rubbish at it because his mind raced around so much. During the session I taught him to take note of his senses in the night and the day as a way of anchoring him to the present moment. I explained that while he couldn't stop his mind from constantly wandering off, he could always choose to gently let go of such distracting thoughts and instead come into the present moment.

After a week of practice he described how being mindful of the touch of his bed on his body in the night had helped to separate himself from his worrisome thoughts. He was amazed how the process of watching them arrive and letting them go, rather than buying into them, had helped to slow down his racing mind and make him feel much more relaxed about being awake in the night.

Starting to Take Notice

Mindfulness, or taking notice of where you are and what you are experiencing right now, involves choosing to be aware of what is going on even if you do not like it. This means noticing the mind and body events that show up when you don't sleep and choosing to make space for them, rather than trying to get rid of or avoid them. It means looking at your insomnia with fresh eyes, as if it is the first time you have ever seen it, rather than through a veil of past judgements. Doing so allows you to act in the most helpful way, as we are encouraged to do by this author.

> Live in the moment,
> Notice what is happening on purpose,
> Choose how you respond to your experiences,
> Rather than being driven by habitual reactions.[3]

I like this quote because it highlights the key aspect of being mindful, which is that you always have a choice as to how you respond to your experiences, and even the most engrained habits, such as buying into unhelpful thoughts or having to take a pill to control your sleep, can be broken if you can see yourself doing it and choose not to.

When you are present, you notice what's really happening. The simple act of noticing yourself struggling with sleep can be very helpful because if you are looking at it, then you are no longer caught up in it.

Have you ever noticed how much easier it is to see other people's problems and offer helpful advice than it is to see your own? Mindfulness offers an outsider's perspective on your own problems, enabling you to respond in the most helpful way to the stress in your life as you experience it.

The tools you are about to learn will help you to see yourself when you're struggling at night or in the day and offer yourself the kind of compassionate support that you would give a friend in need.

To help you achieve this, here are five mindfulness tools for you to start practising now. Each one is designed to build on your own natural mindful ability and provide you with a series of effective tools that can be used during the night and the day. They will only take a few minutes of your time. Before you start, take a moment to read the following three simple guidelines, as they will help your practice in the long term:

◎ **Mindfulness is not designed to get you to sleep.**
When you practise being mindful, it is natural for your mind and body to slow down as you choose to notice everything that is going on moment by moment.

This may make you feel relaxed and even sleepy, and you may notice yourself having the urge to yawn for the first time in a while! Though this is obviously a nice thing to happen, it is important to remember that it is not the aim of mindfulness and using it to control sleep will only push it further away.

○ **Mind-wandering is allowed.** Mindfulness is *not* about having a blank mind. It is perfectly normal for your mind to wander off onto a thought, memory or some other distraction during your practice. If this happens, then gently say, 'Thank you, Mind,' and then return your attention back to whatever you were noticing. It does not matter how many times your mind wanders; what does matter is that you notice when it wanders and that you choose to bring it back.

○ **The time is now.** Aim to practise several times a day. It is possible to practise whenever and wherever you like. You could be walking to work, sitting on a park bench, queuing at the supermarket, cooking dinner or even lying in bed. Simply take the time to notice what you can in that moment.

Exercise: Noticing Your Senses

The aim here is to tune in to your senses as they occur moment by moment.

○ To start, find a comfortable place to sit down or stand, close your eyes and take a moment to get settled.

○ When you are ready, gently bring your awareness

onto your senses, such as what you can hear, feel, smell, taste or, if your eyes are open, what you can see right now in your environment. Simply list everything that you notice either out loud or in your head. For example, 'I can hear a bird,' or, 'I can feel the chair against my back.'

○ Spend about ten seconds focusing on each sense before moving on to the next. If you can't sense something, as for instance there is nothing to smell, then simply report that fact and move on to another sense.

○ If you mind wanders off onto a thought, which it probably will, thank it for the distraction and return your awareness back to noticing your senses.

When to Use?

This exercise can be used anytime and anywhere, day or night – the more practise the better! You can be walking down the street, sat at home or even lying in bed at night. You can do it with your eyes closed or open, and if you fancy a challenge, see if you can notice at least three of each sense before moving on to the next.

Noticing Your Thoughts

We have the capacity to both notice and think about things. However, you may have observed that you spend more time thinking than you do noticing. On a recent holiday I saw an amazing sunset. Unfortunately, as soon as I saw it, I thought that I must take a photo to post on Facebook. As I searched for

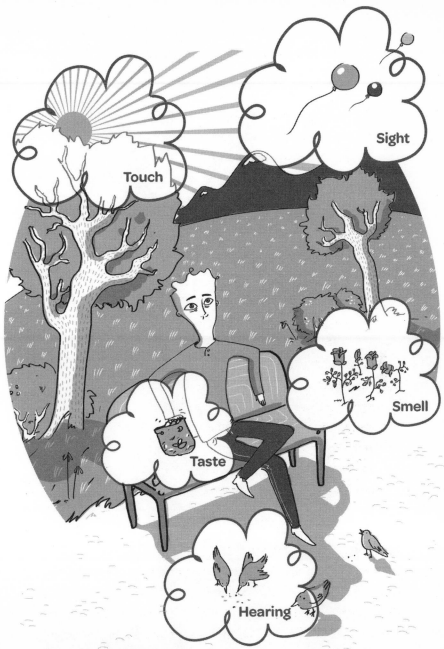

Fig 2.4 Noticing Your Senses

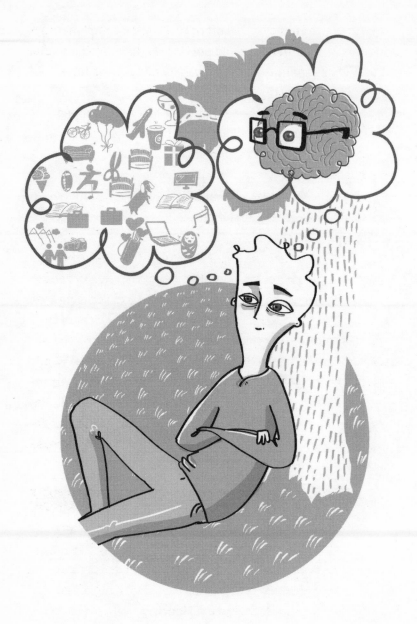

Fig 2.5 **Noticing the Thinker**

my camera, my mind drifted off onto all of the complimentary comments that friends would post when they saw the photo. It took me five minutes to find my camera, by which time I had missed the best of the sunset and did not get the photo! This experience made me realise that I couldn't have stopped myself from having those thoughts and the urge to act upon them, but I could have responded differently to them. In hindsight, if I had acknowledged each thought and then chosen to return my attention back to appreciating the beauty of the sunset in the moment that it gradually dipped below the horizon, I wouldn't have missed it.

Your thoughts can play a key role in how you behave; however, what is vital to remember is that they needn't determine your behaviour. You always have a choice! Realising that there are two of you reading this book at this moment in time can be a strange concept to grasp, but understanding the difference between 'you', the person who is noticing the words on the page, and your 'thinking mind', the person who is thinking about the words on the page, is extremely important. Being able to notice the thinker helps you to realise that you are separate from your thoughts. Let's try the following exercise to demonstrate what I mean.

Exercise: Noticing the Thinker

- Close your eyes for 30 seconds and notice any thoughts or images that pop into your mind.
- As soon as you see a thought or image, say out loud, or under your breath, the word 'thought' and then gently return your attention back to noticing to see if any more pop in.

○ If you like, you can label your thoughts with a descriptive name such as 'work', 'dinner', 'relationship' or whatever they happen to be. If no thoughts turn up, which can sometimes happen, you may find yourself thinking that no thoughts appear to be arriving, which in itself is a thought.

Getting into the habit of looking at your thoughts and labelling them in this way lessens the risk of automatically identifying with your thoughts and getting stuck in them.

Noticing the Judging Mind

So we've seen how we possess the ability to both notice and think about things as they occur. Now we will look at how this can be both helpful and unhelpful. When you take notice, you are simply describing the raw facts as they exist in reality and therefore you are being objective or non-judgemental. For example, if I had stayed to look at the sunset, I would have noticed the different colours and shapes that were formed moment by moment as it set. I would just have noticed and listed what I could see. An important feature of such noticing is that it is based in the here and now, so that if you asked another person what they heard or saw at exactly the same time, they would probably say the same as you.

In contrast, when you are thinking, you are subjective and make a judgement based on past experience and are therefore no longer based in reality. For example, when I saw the sunset, I judged it against every other sunset that I had witnessed in my life and evaluated it to be one of the best that I had ever seen, prompting me to get my camera. This thought was not based on reality, but rather the library of sunsets that I had previously stored in my head. If another person saw it, they could have a completely different opinion based on their own experiences. What is interesting is how this first thought then led me on to other thoughts about how I should take a photo and share it with others, and then even further into the future as to how others might react when they saw the photo. As you can see, with each thought I became further and further removed from reality and more stuck in my own mind.

Understanding the difference between describing and judging is therefore vital when responding to your insomnia. If you are lying in bed awake and you feel your heart beating loudly, what pops into your head? For many insomniacs, the first thing is a judgement such as 'If my heart does not slow down soon, I will not be able to sleep, or, worse, I will have a heart attack!' Obviously such an evaluation is not helpful because it leads to further adrenaline release and therefore further increases in heart rate! It also drives unhelpful behaviour such as trying relaxation strategies to lower it, which if unsuccessful can lead to frustration, more adrenaline, further heart-rate increases and may eventually lead to a panic attack.

In contrast, being able to objectively describe your experiences by saying, 'I can feel my heart beating quickly in my chest,' means that you are accepting what is present at that moment without adding any further unhelpful judgement or emotion to it.

The paradox is that by not trying to change your racing heart rate, you are not adding to it because no more adrenaline is released. A key part of this programme is being able to respond to all of the discomfort that is associated with not sleeping in the day and the night in this mindful and objective way! It may take a bit of practice, but the effects are more far-reaching than just improving your sleep.

'One of my great pleasures is getting out for a long walk as often as I can and this has provided me with a fantastic opportunity to practise mindfulness. In the past, depending on my state of mind I would either have marched purposefully along, lost in my thoughts (usually worrying ones if I was marching) and more or less oblivious to my surroundings but just glad to be out of doors. Or I would have ambled on my way, occasionally pausing to admire the view. Now, being mindful and regardless of the mood I am in, I notice the actual way I walk, the sound of my footsteps and the swinging of my arms. I am more aware of the way I am breathing and am conscious and appreciative of whatever the weather cares to throw at my skin. There is a heightened sense of awareness of all the sights and sounds surrounding me and I look forward to this walking meditation each time I go out.'

Jennifer, London

Noticing Your Breath

The regularity of our breath makes it an excellent anchor to the present moment, and the fact we can do it at any time and it's free makes it a great mindfulness tool. It's also one of the most easily observable bodily sensations, which is why meditators, new and experienced, practise it.

Exercise: Noticing Your Breath

In this exercise you will practise noticing your breath and using it as an anchor to the present moment.

- Find a comfortable chair in a quiet area and sit in a relaxed position with your eyes closed or looking down at the floor.
- Focus your awareness on your breath to observe the physical sensations that occur as you breathe in and out. For example, you might notice movement in your chest or abdominal walls, or you might be able to feel the air rushing in and out of your nose. All you are doing here is noticing what there is to notice when you breathe normally. Aim to settle on noticing one area that you find the easiest to focus on. If it helps, you can also count your breaths, such as saying, 'One,' on the in-breath and, 'Two,' on the out-breath all the way to ten and then starting from one again.
- Resist the urge to change your breath, breathe deeply or see how long you can remain focused on your breath: this is not the aim here.

- As you notice your breath, you may find that your mind has wandered off onto a thought, image, sound or memory that just popped in and momentarily distracted you. When that happens, acknowledge your distraction with a friendly greeting such as 'Hello, Thought' or 'Thank you, Mind' and then gently let go of it by returning your awareness back to your breath.

- Every time your mind wanders off, just keep bringing it back. The aim is to cultivate a gentle relationship with whatever shows up in your mind, even if it is really unhelpful thoughts in the middle of the night.

When to Use?

While practice can be done anywhere or for any length of time, when you first start, find three periods of three minutes in your day: so once in the morning, midday and during the evening. As you progress, you can begin to increase the length of your practice up to ten minutes or more per session, but only if you want to. Your practice can also be performed lying awake at night in bed.

Helpful Tips

Keeping on track. To help you remember to practise, put a note to yourself and stick it somewhere you will see it or set an alarm on your watch or phone. You can also download the Sleep School app that will remind you and log your practice.

No need to compare. Mindful breathing allows you to observe what is present at that moment in time, so comparison between sessions is not necessary and nor does it matter. If your mind starts to judge your sessions, such as 'I was so much better this morning' or 'I am doing really well today because I have no thoughts', then acknowledge these thoughts by thanking your mind for them and then return to your breath.

Self-blame. On first attempts, it is easy to find your 'judging mind' telling you that you are 'doing it all wrong' or that you 'should be feeling more'. If this happens, it is likely that you are actually doing it right because all you are doing is noticing your breath. You are not trying to do special breathing that will enable you to become super relaxed or enter into deep sleep!

Blank canvas. To begin with, you may notice yourself trying to create some form of blank canvas or empty mind because if you could just shut up your mind, then you would be able to sleep. While this may sound like a good idea, it is obviously just falling into the controlling trap again and often just promotes further thoughts. What you are aiming to do is the opposite, meaning that you want to open up your mind, allow a thought to come in, greet it and then gently let go of it and return to your breath.

Letting go. The words 'letting go' can often be misinterpreted as getting rid of your thoughts. It means the same as 'letting be' which is when you choose to allow them to occupy the same space as you and yet you are no longer struggling with them or focused on them. This is why I say that you should 'let go' and then gently return your focus to your breath.

Best intentions. Before starting each practice, take a few moments to notice any intentions that may be lurking in your mind, such as 'I am doing this to relax so that I will fall asleep' or 'I am doing this to get my life back on track.' If such intentions exist in your mind, gently acknowledge them and let them go by focusing on your breath. It is very easy for the judging mind to perceive mindfulness as a tool to help you get to sleep, but it is not. There is no agenda.

Panic feelings. For some of you, even just the thought of focusing on your breath can make you feel breathless. Countless nights of doing deep breathing to get you to sleep or to rid yourself of anxious feelings has left the act of focusing on your breath anchored to feelings of alertness and anxiety! If this is the case for you, then for the time being I would suggest focusing your attention on some other area of your body, such as your heartbeat. Later in the book you will learn tools to get closer to such anxiety and be able to breathe normally once more.

Case Study Continued . . . As part of Carlos's mindfulness practice I decided to teach him mindful breathing. However, as soon as he focused his attention on his breath he reported feeling anxious and wanted to stop. He explained how he had spent countless nights doing deep breathing in the hope of sending himself off to sleep, only to find himself frustrated because it had not worked and some nights made him even more awake. As a result he was very unwilling to use any tools that involved his breath because he knew they would not work for him.

On hearing this, I explained that what he was experiencing was very common. As a result of trying to use deep breathing to force himself to sleep and failing, he had now developed a negative association with breathing. I reminded him that the point of mindfulness was to use the part of his brain that noticed what was going on in the present moment; it was not about relaxing him or getting him off to sleep. I reassured him that I didn't want him to change his breath, but instead just focus on the movement of his breath. In the short term I told him to focus his attention on another regular anchor such as his heartbeat and then with practice start to use his breath.

Noticing Your Sensations and Urges

Every moment of every day your body sends you millions of messages in the form of emotions, sensations and urges about your state of well-being. Whether it is the beat of your heart, the twitch of your muscles or the sensation of feeling hungry, tired, excited or sad, they are all part of the human experience. They provide you with a real-time feed as to what is going on in your body and guide you as to the best way to act in that moment. For example, if we notice we're feeling full while eating, then most of us stop.

Sadly many of us have forgotten how to listen to these feelings or choose to block them out in the hope they will go away, only to have them worsen over time. Sleepless nights can be filled with many unwanted bodily sensations, which is why so many insomniacs go to extreme lengths to avoid sensations they find scary or uncomfortable. Consuming alcohol or drugs can offer short-term peace, but more often than not the sensations come back stronger and shout even louder to get your attention. In the end it can feel like you are at war with your own body. Being willing to listen to, own and make space for your sensations and urges in the moment and recognising that they can't hurt you is a key aspect of being mindful.

Exercise: Noticing Sensations and Urges

○ Find a quiet place to sit, stand or lie and gently close your eyes or direct your gaze ahead of you. For about 10 to 30 seconds notice the sensation of contact between your body and whatever you are sitting, standing or lying on.

○ Move your awareness into your body and take notice of any of the emotions, physical sensations or urges that exist there. Start at your toes and very slowly scan upwards throughout the whole of your body (both sides) until you reach the top of your head. So bring your awareness to your toes, feet, ankles, lower and upper legs, pelvis, abdomen, chest, hands, lower and upper arms, neck and finally your head.

○ Spend 10 to 30 seconds on scanning each area, noticing anything there is to notice, such as a muscle twitch, the beat of your heart, the flutter of your eyelids, butterflies in your tummy, a tightness in your chest, feelings of anxiety or frustration or the urge to move your body, or even nothing. Doing this for five to ten minutes is a good length of time, but it can be done for shorter or longer periods.

○ This is a lovely opportunity to really get to know your body and tap into the life that flows through it. Notice any urges to fight or avoid certain feelings that show up. Be open to welcoming what you notice in an accepting manner even if you don't like it or it feels uncomfortable: 'Hello, Racing Heart' or 'Come on in, Anxious Feelings' or 'Thank you, Urge to Move.'

○ If unhelpful thoughts arrive to try and convince you to avoid experiencing particular sensations, then notice these as well, welcome them and then gently return your attention back to the area you were focused on.

When to Use?

This tool can be done on its own or along with noticing your senses and your breath. At first it can be helpful to scan your bodily sensations in a quiet, relaxing and safe environment. As you become more practised, you can do it anywhere you feel comfortable closing your eyes. Such situations can strengthen the versatility of your practice rather than only being able to be mindful at home when it is calm and quiet. It can also be useful at night if you are awake.

Helpful Tips

Timing. As you progress, you may find that you want to extend it to 10 to 20 minutes or even longer. For a longer session, try lying down in a comfortable place, and if you begin to feel sleepy, then open your eyes and look at the ceiling. You can also do mini body scans lasting only a few seconds, in which you check in with your bodily sensations, such as noticing the beat of your heart while waiting for the kettle to boil.

Night-time. In the middle of the night when you are tired, it's easy to take your unwanted sensations too seriously and immediately try to change, lessen or avoid them. Approach them with playfulness, curiosity and interest, and note how they make you feel and want to react.

Research has shown that mindfulness can be an effective tool to help overcome chronic insomnia. Regular practice has shown to significantly increase the amount of hours spent sleeping, reduce the time taken to fall to sleep and increase sleep efficiency, which is the percentage of time spent in bed actually sleeping. It also improves individual self-recorded insomnia severity scores.[4]

It's believed that this is because mindfulness helps insomniacs to reduce hyper-arousal levels by enabling them to view the arrival of unhelpful thoughts and painful emotions in a less reactive manner, thereby creating more conducive conditions for natural sleep to emerge. Additional research also showed that 8 weeks of mindfulness training in meditation-naïve participants was associated with anatomical changes in the brain regions involved in emotional and cognitive regulation.[5]

The key message is that mindfulness is not designed to get you to sleep, but rather increases your willingness to experience the discomfort associated with not sleeping. When you accept what shows up in the middle of the night, you are less likely to react emotionally and more likely to sleep in the long run.

Mindfulness in Everyday Life

Given how busy life can be sometimes, being mindful – or stopping to smell the roses – can bring a sense of richness to experiences that might otherwise be lost. For this reason mindfulness will not only help you overcome your insomnia, but will also make life richer and more vibrant. And the more you can focus on living your life, the better you will sleep.

Mindfulness has certainly benefited other areas of my own life. When I play with my daughter, my mind is sometimes elsewhere, thinking about things that happened that day or about the next day. In contrast, when I mindfully play with her, every part of me is showing up. I can see her happiness, feel her gentle touch and hear the small changes in her voice. I also note that she knows that I am present and not on Planet Distraction!

Making time for daily noticing practice is great, but it can also be done when you are just getting on with your life, such as going for a mindful walk or eating mindfully.

Exercise: Everyday Mindfulness

Pick an activity that you do every day and focus your attention on it moment by moment as if this is the first time that you have done it. If your mind wanders off, which it probably will do, simply bring it back and continue to notice the activity. Pay attention to each activity for a few days before choosing to focus on another.

When to Use?

Anytime, anywhere. Activities such as brushing your teeth, showering, walking, eating and washing dishes are all good. Boring chores are great, as this is often where your mind will wander the most.

Helpful Tips

Practice reminders. Many daily activities have become so engrained that it can be difficult to remember even to do this practice. A Post-it note on the bathroom mirror can be a helpful reminder for next time you brush your teeth.

Getting stuck. In times of stress or when we feel shattered, it can be really easy to revert back to the old habits of being stuck in your mind or trying to do other things at the same time. Notice that this is happening and come back to focusing solely on the task at hand.

'The Sleep School approach to insomnia totally changed my perspective on sleep. The premise that I might stop trying to "fix" my problem and accept my insomnia instead turned the whole thing on its head. I found the idea that thoughts are just thoughts and that I can choose to observe them, rather than stop them, to be very freeing. The practice of mindful awareness has given me access to an entirely new perspective that not only helped me sleep better but improved my entire life.'

Denise, Vancouver, Canada

Using the Tools at Night

Being mindful at night is about putting you in the right place for sleep but is *not* designed to get you to sleep. It helps you to see your unhelpful struggle with sleeplessness and let go of it, to be present and willing to experience whatever shows up in a non-judgemental manner. It is a helpful response to poor sleep because by choosing to be still and gently take notice, rather than struggle, you are informing your brain that sleeplessness is no longer a threat. You are also saving yourself lots of valuable energy, which will help you to feel more human the next day.

Choosing to be mindful at night does take a lot of courage and willingness because it means removing the blinkers and seeing all of the demons that you have spent so long trying to avoid. For many, it can also mean choosing to stay in bed rather than get up and do things. However, as people who've done this programme already have found, it is never as bad as your thinking mind will make it out to be.

Exercise: Noticing at Night

○ When you first get into bed or if you wake up, it can be helpful to take a few minutes to notice your sense of touch. You can notice the feel of your pillow on your face, the duvet on your toes or where your mattress connects with your body, and if your mind wanders off, you gently return it back. Notice whether the textures are hard, soft, smooth, rough, hot or cold. Touch is a good sensation to start with, since there are not many others to notice at night.

- Now take a few minutes to observe your breath, as above. Remember you can notice your breath in any position and so you can stay in bed.
- Finally, take a few minutes to notice the sensations that arise in your body moment by moment, as detailed in 'Exercise: Noticing Sensations and Urges'.

When to Use?

Practise each of the above mindfulness tools for a few minutes at a time when you go to bed or during the night. Use the tools as a helpful way to let go of your struggles and get you in the right place for sleep, rather than to get yourself to sleep. Remember the normal sleeper who will have a sip of water, go to the toilet, change position and perhaps think of random things when they wake before then falling back to sleep. They don't spend hours on mindful noticing.

Helpful Tips

Lie down. The mindfulness exercises can be done lying in bed in whatever position you find most comfortable. If lying down becomes too much, then a few minutes sitting up or on the edge of the bed can also be an option.

Conserve energy. Take time to enjoy being still and awake in your bed and seek solace in the fact that you are conserving energy for the day ahead.

Wide awake. When choosing to be mindful for the first time in bed, you may feel even more awake. After all, you are choosing to sit with the very demons you have spent many years fighting against and so it is natural to feel even more alert! However, with practice you will notice that despite their best efforts to look scary, they can't actually hurt you and soon you will start to feel relaxed and able to enjoy your bed again.

Moving On

In this week you have learnt to notice what shows up in your mind and body moment by moment. You no longer need to struggle with your insomnia and you may already be benefiting from improved sleep. If this is the case, then I ask you to continue with the five steps, as there is more you can achieve; this is not a quick fix but a lifelong solution to insomnia.

If you are experiencing the opposite, then don't worry, as this is quite normal at this stage. Mindfulness is about being open to experiencing whatever shows up and this can mean pain from your past that is not related to your insomnia. At this stage it can feel like you have opened a can of worms and you wish you hadn't. It is perfectly normal to feel overwhelmed and perhaps even further away from great sleep than when you first started. With continued practice, you will notice a softening of your relationship with your sleeplessness, accompanied by an improvement in your sleep. In the next step you are going to learn some powerful tools that will enable you to welcome any lasting pain and suffering that might be getting in the way of your sleep, so that you can move closer to achieving deep, refreshing sleep every night.

Case Study Continued ... After a couple of weeks Carlos reported that while his sleep had not yet dramatically improved, he felt more relaxed than he had ever been about his sleeplessness and was more able to cope during the day. One big change for him was the amount of energy he now had, which he put down to the fact that he was no longer spending whole nights struggling with his insomnia. This was great as it meant he could start enjoying the more important things in his life, such as spending quality time with his partner and children. Choosing not to struggle at night also helped to send his brain a powerful message that sleep was no longer a threat, something that allowed him to return to a normal sleeping pattern within a couple of months.

WELCOME
...everything that shows up in your mind and your body

'A joy, a depression, a meanness, some momentary awareness comes as an unexpected visitor. Welcome and entertain them all!'

Jelaluddin Rumi

This week we will:

- Find how welcoming all that shows up can bring you closer to natural deep and refreshing sleep every night.
- Understand why your mind and body respond in the way they do to poor sleep and what you can do to help yourself.
- Get to know the unwanted thoughts, emotions, physical sensations and urges that arise in response to not sleeping.
- Learn how to untangle yourself from any unwelcome thoughts you have in your head.
- Begin to feel, create space and play with the emotions, physical sensations and urges that rise and fall in your body in response to poor sleep.

Client Case Study: Mary and Her Racing Mind

Mary had been suffering from insomnia for several years when she visited me at the Sleep Clinic. She described it like being constantly tormented by a gang of monsters who would arrive in her mind and body. At bedtime they would tell her stories about how she was not going to be able to fall to sleep or how tomorrow would be a write-off. The next day they would tell her that everybody thought she looked awful and that she was failing at her job.

Accompanying such thoughts were equally unpleasant feelings of anxiety and sadness, as well as tiredness and nausea. She mentioned that she now believed everything the monsters said and as soon as they arrived she was resigned to the fact that the night would be a write-off, that she would look a mess and that she was going to fail at her job. In her eyes the only way out was to get rid of them because she knew that on the rare occasions when they did not show up, then she could fall to sleep or felt much better the next day.

Welcoming the Unwelcome

This week I want to introduce to you a further revolutionary way of responding to your insomnia that involves harnessing the innate power behind your welcoming response. You will learn how to verbally welcome, move towards, embrace, soften, make space and even play with everything that shows up in your mind and body in the night and the day.

I recognise that being asked to welcome your insomnia might sound a bit bonkers, a step too far or even impossible! It is perfectly normal to feel resentful at the fact that you should be the one to back down or give in to something that has made your life so difficult! However, I am confident that if you continue reading, you will understand how welcoming your insomnia is the key to getting you back to sleep.

Once again, you already possess all of the tools you need because welcoming is a natural part of your everyday life. All you need to do is learn how to apply them to your insomnia so that you can continue on your journey towards achieving good-quality sleep every night.

When you welcome a friend into your home, you move towards them and make eye contact and offer some form of friendly gesture such as a handshake, kiss or verbal welcome. These simple actions are steeped in your evolutionary heritage and are programmed to inform your brain that you are safe! In that moment you become mentally and physically relaxed. Your outlook becomes more positive, your mood lightens, and you have the urge to stay and enjoy the experience. Without knowing it, your level of alertness is also reduced, something that can have a profound effect on your ability to sleep. Take a moment now to think about how you respond to your insomnia and what sort of message you think this is sending to your brain.

Night-Time Battles

If you are anything like many of my clients, the act of going to sleep could be likened to going into battle, one with inevitable results. Unfortunately, what you put in is generally what you get out, and sleep is no exception to the rule! Any attempts to fight, avoid, change or get rid of experiencing your insomnia tell your brain that you are being threatened, triggering your innate survival response. In this moment you become mentally and physically alert as your brain prepares you to stand

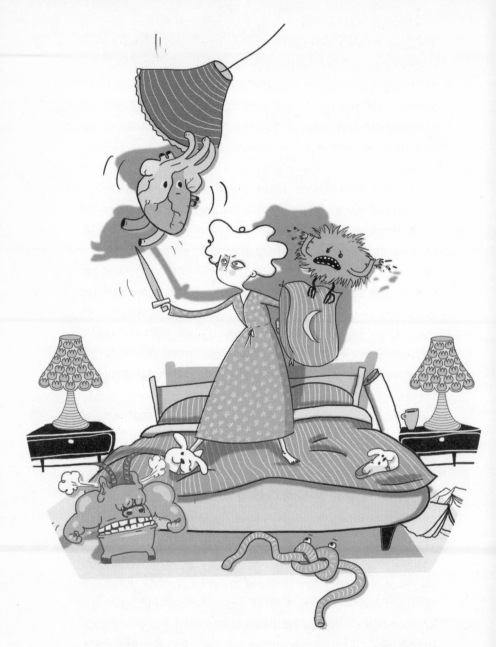

Fig. 3.1 **Bedroom Battles**

and fight or withdraw in flight. Your mind begins to race with thoughts, your mood darkens, your muscles tense, your body shrinks, and you become wide awake. How you choose to respond towards your insomnia therefore determines your insomnia, and only by learning to welcome it can you retrain your brain to sleep soundly once more.

Case Study Continued . . . Mary asked me to show her how to banish the monsters because everything she had tried had failed. I said I would love to be able to make her thoughts and feelings go away, but it was not possible and, if anything, would further fuel their strength and numbers! Instead I proposed the concept of actually allowing them to exist and welcoming them. In doing so, her brain would instantly learn that such thoughts and feelings were not enemies that needed to be attacked and that it was safe for her to sleep. Responding in this way also meant that such thoughts and feelings no longer took centre stage, plaguing her night and day.

Over time Mary learnt that while she couldn't control when they showed up or what they said, she could control how she responded to the monsters and welcoming them was the most helpful response. Most importantly, she realised the monsters didn't have to go away for her to be able to lie in bed relaxed, be able to fall asleep or to be able to get on with her work the next day.

In the next section you will learn a series of unique tools designed to welcome all of the unwanted thoughts that show up in the night and day in response to not sleeping. In doing so, you will join the many clients who have successfully used the welcome response to calm their racing minds and anxious feelings and achieve great sleep every night.

'After a bit of trial and error, I discovered that the techniques which were most helpful to me were the simplest ones. So as I started to notice myself having unhelpful thoughts, I would just say, "I'm having a thought about sleep again," or, "I'm having a thought about the rest of my life." The ones that were most common I would start to abbreviate and even own: "I'm having my sleep thought" or "my forever thought". I would also welcome them: "Hello, Sleep Thought. You're here again." Over time and with recovery and practice, I have found that I don't even need to give my thoughts this much attention if I don't want to. These days when I notice myself brooding about anything (not necessarily related to sleep), once I become aware of it, I am able to just go, "Oh, I'm thinking again," and kind of acknowledge to myself that it's not even real. I then come back to the present moment of my life, usually by focusing on the immediate physical sensations that I can feel and maybe what I can hear and see.'

Alice, London

Monsters in Your Head

When you are trying to fall to sleep, there is nothing more annoying than a racing mind preventing you from doing so. Like Mary, it can feel like your mind becomes home to a gang of little monsters who arrive from nowhere as soon as your head hits the pillow. Intent on keeping you awake, they eagerly jump from solving your life problems to churning through old memories, then running through the events of the day and

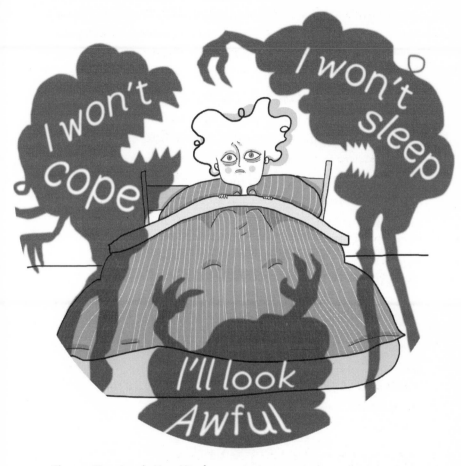

Fig. 3.2 **Monsters in Your Head**

revisiting conversations or just filling your head with a catchy tune! They can also become catastrophe analysts, relentlessly going over questions such as 'Why did my poor sleep start?', 'How am I going to fix it?' and 'What will happen if I don't sleep?', all of which keep you wide awake.

Listening to these thoughts night after night, it can be tough not to believe them to be reality. Much like when you buy into a good book, film or daydream, you are caught in a trance-like state in your own mind. The only difference is that the stories in your head typically can't be put down or switched off so easily!

In that moment fighting, avoiding or trying to change your thoughts can feel like the only options available to you, but doing so brings them back stronger and in greater numbers! Welcoming them can therefore have the opposite effect, but before you learn how to do this, you must understand why your mind thinks this way in the first place. In reality, hard as it may be to believe, your mind is actually just trying to protect you!

Our Survival Response

In evolutionary terms you are more likely to be able to survive if your mind is constantly active and always trying to predict what could go wrong. This explains why the bulk of your fifty thousand or so thoughts a day appear negatively charged. Your brain is permanently monitoring what is going on in the present moment and relating it to information from your past that might be similar and of use in the future.

You have probably experienced this when you've heard a meaningful song on the radio and you've been transported back to the time you first heard it. The smell of freshly cut grass does it for me – taking me back to hot summer days spent playing in the garden as a child.

From a survival perspective, this was a hugely effective process, as it managed to use past experiences to predict potential threats in the future. This explains why when you encounter anything to do with sleep, be it the act of going to bed, being awake in the night, feeling anxious or even just reading a newspaper article about sleep, your brain can't help but refer back to your own sleepless memories and extrapolate accordingly.

This explains why if you find yourself awake in the night, your mind can become filled with memories of past poor sleep and catastrophic predictions of future sleeplessness. Typically they start with the generic question of 'Why am I awake?' which is then later followed by thoughts such as 'What can I do to get myself back to sleep?', 'Should I take a pill?' or 'Should I get up and do something?' If your actions don't appear to work, then thoughts such as 'It does not seem to be working', 'How many hours have I got left?' or 'What is wrong with me?' begin to creep in.

As time ticks on, your thoughts start to predict the future, such as 'I won't be able to cope tomorrow' or 'I will look awful.' If poor sleep continues, it is normal for your mind to look for ways to end your pain and suffering and thoughts of suicide can arise for people with long-term insomnia.

SLEEP FACT

Thought challenging is a widely used approach to combat negative thoughts. For example, on going to sleep if you notice yourself having the thought 'I will not sleep tonight', you might choose to challenge its validity based on your past experience and replace it with a more positive thought, such as 'I have had a couple of good nights this week and so there is a chance that I might sleep well tonight.' At face value, giving your thoughts a more rational and balanced outlook does make sense and should help to quell the rising levels of anxiety and promote better sleep. However, in my work I've noticed this is not always the case.

One of the main issues is that most people simply do not believe the rational statements they are saying to themselves, especially in the middle of the night. Many also find the process to be like an endless tug of war in which their minds create a thought and then they challenge it, as if they are constantly tugging back and forth.

Another potential problem is the fact that challenging thoughts places an unhealthy level of importance on something that at its most basic level is just a bit of noise in your head. The act of challenging therefore unhelpfully glorifies or sensationalises the unhelpful thought, rather than just accepting it as a thought. Also, most insomniacs complain that they already have too many thoughts in their head and challenging them only leads to more.

Another issue is that thought challenging often uses past experience to predict the future in a positive way. For example, 'I have had two good nights out of four, so there is a chance I might sleep well again tonight.' While it can be helpful to be aware of any positive sleep history such as the fact that you may have managed to get some sleep, ultimately you can't predict the future and doing so can be a dangerous business. You may feel upset when your predictions do not turn out the way you want them to and as a result feel you are back to square one. In the end it is vital to remember that the past has been and gone, while the future has not happened. Focus on what shows up in the present moment and choose the thoughts you buy into and let go of the ones that you don't.

Trying to suppress your thoughts is equally troublesome, with research showing that it can fuel the very thoughts you are trying to avoid as well as the emotional response connected to them.[6]

Welcoming Your Unwelcome Thoughts

When you welcome your thoughts, you can look at them and put them into context. You respect the fact that they are a product of your mind, but you have the mental clarity not to take them as the literal truth. You no longer need to struggle to get rid of them or change them into something more positive, but rather accept them for the bits of noise or objects that just so happen to have arrived in your head in this moment. Most importantly, welcoming enables you to respond to your unwanted thoughts in a way that does not fuel further thoughts or wakefulness.

To be able to welcome your unwelcome thoughts, first it helps to get to know what turns up. This may be an easy process as you see them show up every day, but if you've had years of repetition, they may be automatic and you only know they've been because you suddenly feel anxious or experience a racing heart rate.

Here is a list of some of the common thoughts that insomniacs report having about their insomnia and the effect it has on their lives. I have given each one a short hand descriptive nickname or label. This can be a quick way of referring to them, which you will use later. For now take a look and identify which ones sound like yours and start to make a list of your own including giving them shorthand names.

Think about the stories, comments, put-downs and so on that you repeat to yourself in the night and the day. If your thoughts are mostly images then have a go at drawing the scenes or describe how they look.

You could try writing your thoughts down on paper which helps to get them out of your head and create some physical separation between you and them. Write only in the daytime as normal sleepers don't write out long lists of their thoughts in the night. Once you have a list, you may find it helpful to keep it near you to remind you that you are separate from them.

THOUGHT NAME	THOUGHT
Sleep	I won't sleep tonight
Coping	If I don't sleep tonight I won't be able to cope tomorrow
Fix it	What can I do to fix my sleep?
Medication	Should I take another pill?
Why?	Why is this happening to me?
What if?	What if I don't sleep tomorrow night as well?
Failure	I'm a failure because I can't sleep
Bully	I need to stop being so pathetic and sort myself out
Self judgment	Why am I doing this to myself?
Health	This must be seriously affecting my health
Time	How long have I got left to sleep?
Lonely	I'm the only person who can't sleep
Jealousy	It's not fair, why can they sleep and I can't?
Prop	If I don't wear my ear plugs then I won't be able to sleep
Noise	If he starts snoring then I won't be able to sleep

Bed sharing	I won't be able to sleep if I share a bed
Tiredness	If I don't sleep soon I will be shattered tomorrow
Function	If I don't sleep I won't be able to perform to my best
Looks	I will look awful tomorrow
Feeling	I will feel wretched tomorrow
Work	I am not able to do my job anymore
Other people	Everyone will think that I am on drugs
Wind down	I need to be relaxed to get to sleep
Resigned	I will never sleep properly again
Sabotage	What if poor sleep returns?
Depression	I am going to become depressed
Anxiety	If I feel anxious then I won't sleep
Racing heart	If my heart beats any faster I will have a heart attack
Relationship	This is affecting my relationships
Approach	This approach won't work for me
Life	This is stopping me from living my life

Case Study Continued . . . To explain to Mary how she had attached meaning to her monsters' thoughts, I used a common ACT metaphor known as 'Milk, Milk, Milk'. For this, I asked her to think about the word 'milk' and describe what popped into her mind, which was that it was cold, white, creamy and that it comes from cows and is delivered in a carton. I explained that these were the associations that she had developed over time in connection with this word and for others it would differ. I then asked her to rapidly repeat the word out loud for one minute and notice what happened. She reported that the word lost its meaning and in the end became just a strange noise that bore no resemblance to the original associations. She was amazed to see how such a long-standing belief could become just noises and began to realise that perhaps she didn't need to get rid of her monsters after all.

Exercise: Welcoming Your Thoughts

Here are a few different ways to practise welcoming your thoughts:

Welcoming. Whenever you notice an unwelcome thought pop into your head, greet it in a friendly manner: 'Welcome', 'Come on in' or 'Good to see you!' If they are a regular guest, acknowledge this by saying, 'You again,' or, 'Good to see you again.' Then return your attention back to whatever you were doing just before the thought arrived (e.g. lying in bed).

Describing. If the thought of welcoming is too much too soon, then you can acknowledge your guests in a neutral manner instead. When they arrive, prefix them with a descriptive sentence such as 'I am having the thought that if I don't sleep, I won't be able to cope.' Alternatively you can describe what your mind is doing, such as 'There goes my mind babbling on again' or 'I've heard this story before.' Doing this creates much-needed distance between you and your thoughts.

Thanking. 'Thank you, Mind, for this thought' is another simple, effective and compassionate way of untangling yourself from your thoughts. This separates you from your thoughts and tells your brain that you are safe.

Naming. As you become more familiar with your thoughts, you can start to use their shorthand names and be playful in your approach, such as 'Just got into bed and I see that the classic Sleep, Pill, Coping and Looks thoughts have all turned up, and I see you've brought Anxiety and Frustration along for the ride too! Welcome, everyone.'

Play with your thoughts. Some thoughts will sound very convincing and therefore difficult to untangle yourself from, especially in the night. In this case you can sing to them (e.g. 'Happy Birthday') or use a comic voice (e.g. Homer Simpson), either in your head or out loud. This can make them sound a little silly and less believable. Or you could try changing the tempo or pitch of your thoughts. Anything that distorts how they sound in your head can be enough to break the associations that keep you tangled up in them.

When to Use?

Practise welcoming your thoughts in the day and the night. The more daytime practice you can get, the easier it will be to shrug off night-time thoughts.

Helpful Tips

The goal. Welcoming your thoughts is not to get rid of them or change their content, but to untangle yourself from them. You can then let go of holding them in your awareness by returning your attention back to whatever else you were doing. In the night this could mean being still and calm in bed and mindfully noticing the touch of your pillow on your face.

Images. If your thoughts tend to be mostly images, such as you picture yourself lying awake all night panicking or not being able to cope at work the next day, then playing with the functional quality of the images also works to break the formed associations. For example, try putting them on a cinema screen or changing the size, colour, shape and speed of the pictures as they pass through your head.

Creating distance. You may notice that by prefixing thoughts with a short descriptive sentence you create some distance between you and them. It also acts to slow down the thought, enabling you to access the rational part of your brain that knows it is your choice whether you buy into your thought or not.

In the next section you will learn tools for welcoming all of the unwanted emotions, physical sensations and urges that show up in the night and day in response to not sleeping.

Fearing the Feeling

Your emotional reactions and physical sensations are an evolutionary survival mechanism that prepare you to run away from danger or move towards safety. They can be short-lived and intense, like the urge to run when someone jumps out and scares you or the feelings of warmth when reunited with an old friend. They can also be long-lasting, such as experienced during love and grief.

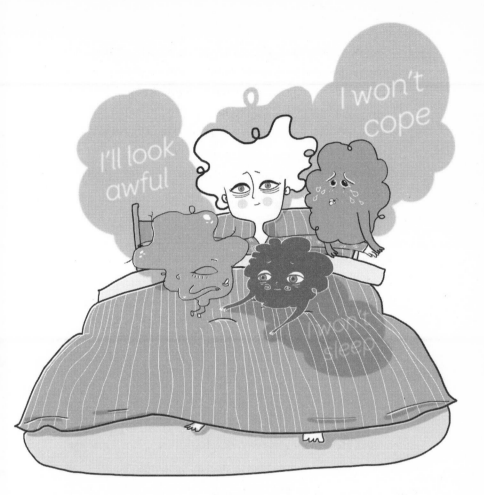

Fig. 3.3 **Welcoming Your Unwelcome Thoughts**

We experience the ebb and flow of these sensations as they respond to life events 24 hours a day. This explains how you can go from feeling happy and jubilant to anxious and angry in a matter of seconds. It only takes the arrival of some sad news or even just a sad thought to pop into your head to completely change your emotional and physical landscape. They are the product of chemical reactions occurring in your brain and body, and as a result are out of your control. However, this lack of control is mutual because while they may incline you to act in a certain way, they do not con-

> Insomnia affects the way you feel both emotionally and physically, and affects how you behave.

trol how you eventually behave. For example, when going for an interview, you may feel scared and have the urge to run away, but it is your choice whether you do or not.

The link between poor sleep and being able to regulate our emotions has even made its way into our daily sayings. This is why we playfully quip, 'Looks like someone got out of the wrong side of bed this morning,' when someone is in a bad mood, or describe a small child as being 'over-tired' if they start to become emotional or easily upset.

When it comes to insomnia, the range of emotional reactions and physical responses that you can experience is vast and individual. If my sleep is disrupted even for one night, a host of new arrivals show up in my mind and body the next day. Feelings of irritation, annoyance and grumpiness, as well as hunger, sugar cravings and tiredness all arrive. For some people, it can cause them to feel sad, hyper, edgy and anxious.

The most common arrival is the feeling of anxiety, or a knot in the stomach, when you realise that it is nearly time to go to bed. On going to bed, you might start to notice your heart or breathing rate quickens, especially if you don't fall to sleep in good time. This often leads to feelings of frustration, helplessness or resignation, especially if it is a regular occurrence. At this moment you feel overwhelmed with the urge to toss and turn or get up and do things rather than lie in bed wide awake.

As time passes, anger can show up and be directed towards anyone or anything. Partners, pillows, noisy neighbours and work colleagues can all bear the brunt of your tiredness-fuelled rage. A feeling of jealousy is also very common, especially if you happen to sleep next to someone who falls to sleep as soon as their head hits the pillow! Over time feelings of sadness, hopelessness, loneliness and depression can appear and drain you of your zest for life. For some, such feelings can sometimes be the tip of the iceberg and, if allowed, can bring to the surface deeper, darker emotions relating to past experiences.

For me, a few poor nights can bring past fears of failure into the present with such strength that it feels like they never left. For others, it opens the door to old feelings of depression, rejection, anxiety and guilt, to name but a few. In this way sleeplessness has the power to reconnect you to your unwanted emotional past and so it makes sense that you would wish to do all you can to get rid of it. However, much like your thoughts, you have little control over the way you feel and trying to control feelings often only worsens them. By contrast, learning to welcome them offers a powerful way of resetting your emotional thermostat, allowing you to sleep soundly at night.

SLEEP FACT

Recent research has been able to identify the link between tiredness and emotional regulation. It would appear that sleep deprivation inhibits your ability to regulate your mood or cope with everyday emotional

challenges. Effectively you revert to a more primitive
state, whereby your amygdala goes into overdrive,
exacerbating your emotional responses beyond the level
required for the situation.[7] This could explain why so
many of my clients report experiencing such excessive
emotional responses in the middle of the night or the
next day, with the smallest of events triggering an
unexpected outpouring of tears or acts of aggression.
Tiredness has also been shown to affect the processing
of your memories, with research suggesting that sleep-
deprived individuals find it easier to recall unpleasant
memories over more happy ones.[8]

The failure to regulate one's emotional system may
also explain why poor sleep is so often accompanied by
additional psychological disorders, such as anxiety and
depression. Traditionally, insomnia has been seen as a
symptom of depression; this is why many of my clients
are still told that they are depressed and are treated for
that rather than insomnia. However, research shows
that insomnia can be both a symptom and cause for
depression.[9] This makes sense because if you do not
sleep, your mood is lowered and you are more likely
to feel depressed. It also explains why so many of my
clients report that if they do get a good night, their
mood is significantly elevated.

Learning to mindfully look at and welcome your
emotions and sensations and untangle yourself from
them in the middle of the night or the next day is
therefore one way to address the relative imbalance
created by sleep loss.

Case Study Continued . . . After a month of practice Mary mentioned that when she went to bed, she now imagined she was a headmistress at a primary school and that the pupils were her monsters. She described how she would take a class register to see who was attending each night and found it incredibly helpful because in doing so, she no longer feared the monsters and actually looked forward to seeing who was going to be present. She was amazed to find that while she was not trying to get rid of them, the number of attendees had actually fallen since doing the practice. However, she did notice that if she had something on the next day that would require her to be on form, the classroom filled up again. But this time she was willing to register them for her so-called 'night school' and recognised that she could even fall to sleep with a full classroom. After a while she even decided to drop the 'monster' description, as she no longer saw them in this way.

Welcoming Your Unwelcome Emotional Reactions, Physical Sensations and Urges

As with your thoughts, the first step towards untangling yourself from your emotional reactions and sensations is to familiarise yourself with them. One of the most common emotions that shows up for clients in the night and the day is anxiety, which often manifests itself as a racing heart, which might urge the client to do relaxation. Likewise, if you feel fear, you might experience muscle tension and have the urge to take pills. A sense of desperation might cause a tight chest and cause you to have the urge to drink alcohol. Or if you feel bored, the resulting restlessness might give you the urge to get up and do something.

Now think about your insomnia and start to make a list of your own. For example, you might write, 'Lonely – knot in stomach – wake up partner,' or, 'Frustration – adrenalised – scream and shout.' Feel free to add any that I haven't mentioned: this is about *you* getting to know *your* insomnia. As you do it, you may start to feel a little uncomfortable, scared and even have the urge to stop. This is perfectly normal. You probably felt something similar on your first day of school or when you started a new job. If it happens, take a moment to acknowledge who is showing up in your body right now, offer them a friendly welcome and then carry on with the job. It is important to remember that while you can't control which emotions and sensations show up in the night, you can always choose how you respond to them. In the next section you will learn techniques to use on your journey to becoming a good sleeper again.

Exercise: Welcoming Your Emotional Reactions, Physical Sensations and Urges

Here are some ways to welcome your unwelcome emotions, physical sensations and urges that show up at night or during the day:

Meet and greet. As you did with your unwelcome thoughts, when you notice the arrival of any emotions, physical sensations or urges, offer them a friendly welcome, such as 'Hello, Frustration, good to see you this evening' or 'Greetings, Urge to Take a Pill' or 'Welcome, Tiredness. I see you've decided to join me today.' Being light-hearted in this way prevents you getting unhelpfully caught up in them and amplifying them further.

Describe. Take a moment to non-judgementally describe all of the emotions, physical sensations and urges that occur in your body. Imagine that they are objects within you and you are 'looking at' them. To assist your objectivity, scan your body answering the following questions as you go:

- **Which emotions are showing up?** For example, 'I can sense anxiety and panic.'
- **Which physical sensations are showing up?** For example, 'I can sense my heart beating and a knot in my stomach.'
- **Where do you feel them most strongly and weakly in your body?** For example, 'They are strongest in the pit of my tummy and weakest in my toes.'
- **Are they on the surface or deep inside of you?** For example, 'They are deep in the centre of my tummy.'
- **What are they doing?** For example, 'They are spinning round very fast.'
- **Do they have any shape, form or colour?** For example, 'They look like a big, tight, tangled ball of rope that is on fire.'
- **Do they have any weight, texture or temperature?** For example, 'They feel very heavy, rough and hot.'

Make space. Allow your emotions, physical sensations and urges to exist within you by creating a space for them to live. Taking your answers from the previous questions (for example, 'They look like a big, tight, tangled ball of rope that is on fire'), use your imagination to create a large space (as big as you want) around them and within you. Allow them to move freely and float within the space. If you want, you can then bring your breath into the space to help create that sense of openness and freedom, and a softening of your relationship with them. Take time to observe them as they move around the space and notice how it feels to allow them to exist within you, rather than constantly struggling to squeeze them out.

Play. Once you are familiar with them and can see them as being separate from you, you can start to play with them in your mind. Take a moment to give them a physical character. Imagine being sat in the audience at the theatre looking at them as they come out one by one onto the stage. Dress them in playful clothes and make them act according to their characters, such as an angry bull charging around the stage with steam coming out of its ears.

Floating. Take a moment to float with your urges as they rise and fall during the night and day. Run through every detail of your experience in your mind and be as objective as possible, such as 'I feel the urge to get up and take another pill', 'My mind is filling with "Pill" thoughts', 'My body is becoming restless' or 'I feel a rising level of anxiety in my body.' Notice how despite not feeling very nice, you can float with these urges and

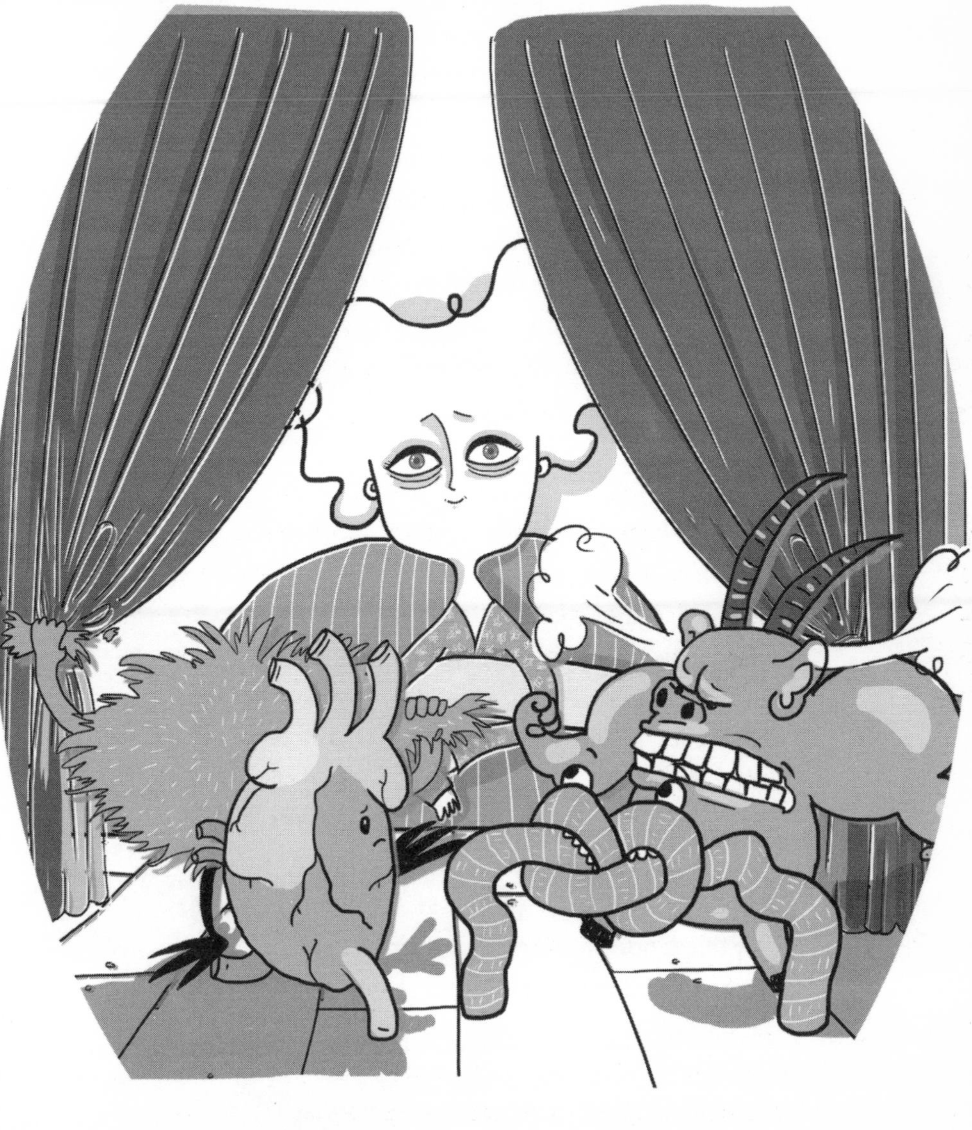

Fig. 3.4 **Playing with Your Emotions, Sensations and Urges**

experiences and choose how you want to behave rather than become consumed by them.

When to Use?

You can practise welcoming your emotions, physical sensations and urges anytime they show up in the night or the day. If they only show up at night, then you could start practising during the day by recalling a recent poor night and welcoming all the sensations as they arrive in your memory.

Helpful Tips

Feel your feelings. The point of this tool is to feel your emotions, physical sensations and urges for what they really are, rather than fearing what they are not. This reduces the chance of amplifying them further and allows you to get back to being in bed awake and hopefully falling to sleep sooner rather than later. Having said this, the tool is not designed to get rid of, lessen or change them in any way, but this can happen when you open yourself up to experiencing them. If your sensations disappear quickly, then so be it, but remember that this is not the purpose of the tool, and if used with such an intention in the future, it might not have the same result.

Stronger at night. Most clients report that the sensations are strongest either when they are going to bed or in the middle of the night. If this is the case, then it can

be helpful to practise the exercise during the day to prepare you for sitting with your sensations at night. Sensations often feel worse at night simply because there
are no distractions as there are during the day.

Welcome thoughts. As you perform this tool, it is common for your thinking mind to send you a constant
stream of worrisome thoughts such as 'This is awful' or
'What can I do to make it go away?' Welcoming such
thoughts will help to keep you on track rather than
heading back to the quick fixes!

Energy efficiency. Take note of how much energy you
are putting into trying to get rid of your unwanted sensations rather than allowing them to simply be. You
may find that you have been expending 100 per cent of
your energy without even knowing it.

Describing versus evaluating. As you perform this exercise, it is very easy to become overwhelmed and move
from describing mode into evaluating. Please note that
'to describe' means 'to give an objective and non-judgemental account of what is happening at that moment'.
For example, 'I am feeling the sensation of my heart
beating fast in my chest.' Whereas 'to evaluate' means
'to give a subjective and judgemental opinion of your
experiences'. For example, 'My heart is beating so fast
that I think I am having a heart attack!' Learning to describe your experiences mindfully in this way helps you

to see your sensations for what they are and realise that while they might be uncomfortable, they can't actually hurt you. When looking at your emotions and sensations, it can be helpful to remind yourself of this fact by asking yourself, 'Are they hurting me, or are they uncomfortable?'

Trigger points. It is common for many emotional and physical sensations to occur in response to a specific trigger such as moving to the bedroom, lying down on the pillow, waking up in the middle of the night or knowing that you have to get up early for a meeting. Getting to know such triggers can allow you to be mindfully prepared and willing to experience whatever shows up.

Full to the brim. Sometimes when you create a space, the imagined objects can appear to grow in size and fill the space. If this happens, then gently observe it with curiosity and interest. If you want to, you can increase the size of the space with your imagination.

Urge to block it out. If you feel the urge to block the object out or your judging mind keeps instructing you to get rid of it, then simply thank your body for the urge and your mind for the thoughts and come back to creating the space. The act of allowing sensations space shows that you are willing to experience them and that you no longer fear them.

Playfully experience. Giving your emotions and physical sensations playful characters helps to objectify them and therefore enhance your willingness to get closer to and experience them. Please be aware that it is not designed to mask or avoid them in any way.

SLEEP FACT

Discussing our problems with others has been the antidote for human suffering since time began. Whether it is talking to other members of your clan, chatting to a friend over coffee or even telling your woes to a Guatemalan worry doll, it would appear that a problem shared is a problem halved. However, it is only recently that we have been able to unlock the therapeutic power that comes from describing our feelings.

Recent research demonstrates that when you can describe your emotions, you diminish the response of your amygdala and limbic system, the areas of your brain that produce the emotional distress.[10] The act of describing activates the rational part of your brain known as your prefrontal cortex, which then assesses whether the current emotional response is helpful or not and controls it accordingly.

This suggests that learning to defuse your thoughts, emotions and physical sensations by objectively describing them in your head or out loud could be likened to the therapeutic power that comes from discussing your problems with a good friend or therapist. Choosing to use such techniques at known

> times of heightened stress, such as when you go to bed,
> wake up in the middle of the night or the next day,
> could therefore enable you to respond in the most
> helpful way to poor sleep.

Case Study Continued . . . Something that Mary really struggled with was daytime tiredness. She described how some days she felt so wretched and tired that she could not concentrate at work and kept forgetting things. She questioned whether she really needed to accept such awful feelings in order to be able to sleep properly and whether she would ever feel normal again. I explained to her that while not sleeping may make her feel awful the next day, struggling with it only made the feelings a lot worse. I reminded her of the tug-of-war metaphor and how the harder she pulled against her insomnia, the stronger it pulled back. More importantly, though, it also fuelled her level of nocturnal wakefulness because she would spend all night thinking about how bad she would feel the next day. I asked her to get to know her daytime sensations in the same way she had done at night.

A few weeks later she reported that whenever she noticed a sensation, she would offer it a friendly greeting, such as 'Hello, Tiredness' or 'Thanks for turning up today, Knackered.' She described how when they were really strong, she would picture them one by one coming out along a conveyor belt, like the prizes on an old game show that she used to watch. As each one arrived, she would shout out what it was and actually began to look forward to who was going to show up next. She was amazed at how just noticing 'tiredness' rather than struggling with it avoided amplifying it. She also reported that since adopting this approach, she no longer worried about how she was going to feel if she didn't sleep, which meant that she slept well most of the time. Plus, even if she did have a poor night, she said that she would simply get on with her day to the best of her ability and allow the tiredness to come along for the ride.

BUILD
...your new sleeping pattern

*'Sleeping is no mean art: for its sake
one must stay awake all day'*

Friedrich Nietzsche

This week we will:

- Learn what normal sleep is, how much your body needs and when is the best time for you to be getting it.
- Discover how sleep is made up of different stages that repeatedly cycle and change throughout the night.
- Understand how important it is to regulate your sleep when building a new and long-lasting sleeping pattern that fits in with the rest of your life.
- Learn what normal sleepers do to get a good night's sleep and start to behave like one.

'I had seen several doctors including sleep doctors and found no relief from CBT or their other suggestions and the medications offered. It was very frustrating. Until I found The Sleep School's programme, I thought something irreparable had happened to my sleep drive and I would have insomnia for the rest of my life. Their explanation enabled me to gain some perspective on my insomnia. The programme doesn't require any major changes or adaptations to your life. It's easy to implement, and once you get the hang of it, it really is so helpful for improving your sleep. Some of the exercises are good to practise for daily life stressors as well.

'It's been a year since starting the programme and I am happy to say that I sleep pretty darn well. Instead of the two, three, four hours of broken sleep that I used to have, I am sleeping about seven hours per night and more on the weekends!'

Lori, Colorado

Biological processes in your brain work together to regulate your sleep. Sleep is an automatic process that we can't control; by that I mean we can't fall asleep just because we want to. Having said that, it's very easy to disturb your natural sleep rhythm, as we see with insomnia. To help rebuild a normal sleeping pattern, we want to give you the best possible chance of finding a rhythm that suits your natural tendencies and fits with your life. In order to do this, we will help you to understand:

- what normal sleep is
- how long you should sleep

- what time of day you should sleep
- how to behave like a normal sleeper.

What Is Normal Sleep?

When you suffer from insomnia, you might think that eight hours of unbroken, refreshing sleep is the ideal. It might help you to have some clarity about what normal sleep is and the variations that can exist, so you can create a realistic expectation of good sleep.

There are no two people in the world who have the same night's sleep, nor will you experience the same night's sleep twice. There will always be variations and wakings in each night. Nor is there such thing as a perfect night's sleep: everyone takes a short time to fall asleep and wakes one or more times a night. As we've said throughout the programme, it is how we behave when we can't get to sleep and what we do when we wake that makes us either a normal sleeper or an insomniac.

Sleep is measured by placing electrodes on the head to detect the brain's electrical activity from which it can be seen whether you are awake or asleep. An entire night of recording for a normal adult sleeper is shown on the sleep hypnogram that follows. It highlights the repeated cycles between wakefulness, light, deep and then rapid eye movement (REM) sleep that occur in a typical night of sleep.

Looking at the graph, you will be surprised to see that light sleep is the most common sleep stage, accounting for at least 50 per cent of a normal sleeper's night. When you are in this state, you tend to feel drowsy and are gently beginning to lose your grasp on the external world before falling into deep sleep.

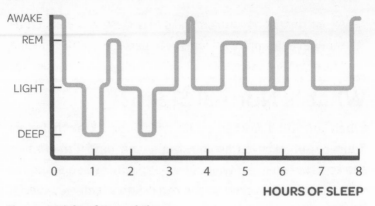

Fig. 4.1 **A Night of Normal Sleep**

As the name suggests, this is the deepest type of sleep, which explains why when you wake up out of it, you can feel disorientated. It's in deep sleep that the body grows and repairs itself, so it's absolutely essential. You may be surprised again to learn that even normal sleepers only spend around 20 per cent of the night here, and most of this is achieved within the first third of the night.

The final stage of sleep is REM, which occurs in the latter part of the night and early hours of the morning until you wake. During this stage your brain is very active, laying down memory, managing your emotions from the day and dreaming, which tends to make it light and increases your chance of being easily woken. This also explains why you might wake up remembering your dreams or feeling shattered and unrefreshed in the morning.

You sleep in cycles that are an hour and a half to two hours long, and at the end of each one you will experience a small awakening before starting the next. Most normal sleepers will have on average between four and five cycles and therefore awakenings per night, although many will be completely unaware of them. Good-quality sleep is measured by the number of complete sleep cycles you achieve rather than single sleep stages slept.

These awakenings allow you to change your body position in order to prevent aches and pains, as well as offering an opportunity for you to go to the toilet. If you are elderly, this could explain why your sleep is more broken now than when you were younger.

It is also thought that the constant awakenings are an evolutionary protective mechanism designed to allow you to sleep and yet still wake up at regular intervals to check for any approaching danger. If you think about it, human survival has depended on wakefulness, which is why you can be ready to fight or take flight in a fraction of a second and yet it takes a normal sleeper at least 15 minutes to fall to sleep.

While you no longer have to worry about being eaten by a sabretooth tiger, you do have worries, which to your primitive brain are just as deadly and worthy of either waking you up from sleep or keeping you awake to be on guard. This explains why the more you struggle to get yourself to sleep, the more you tap into your evolutionary past and the more you wake yourself up. One of the aims of this book is to respond skilfully to such awakenings, training your brain that it is safe to repeatedly experience sleep cycle after sleep cycle without needing to consciously wake you up or keep you awake.

Client Case Study: John and His Night-Time Activity

John had been suffering from insomnia on and off for twenty years, ever since he left school and started work. By the time he came to see me, he was stuck in a lot of unhelpful habits, such as spending too long trying to sleep, constantly getting out of bed if he couldn't sleep and sleeping in the spare room away from his partner. In coming to see me, he hoped that I would help him to sleep through the night in the same bed as his wife.

How Long Should I Sleep?

It is common for insomniacs to spend longer in bed than they actually need to in the hope of increasing the chance of getting more sleep. The simple fact is that spending too long in bed can have the opposite effect and reduce the quality of your sleep. You want to be in bed for the number of hours your body needs to sleep and no longer.

While the average amount of sleep that an adult human needs is seven to eight hours, the range is between four and ten hours. How much sleep you need is therefore a very individual thing, and needing more or less than others is not a problem, just as long as you are getting enough to wake up feeling relatively refreshed and able to function during the day.

I realise that you may not be at this point yet, but setting the right sleep duration for your individual needs will help you to get there. To work out how much sleep you could expect to achieve and thus how much time to stay in bed take a look at the following:

1   **Requirement for your age** – The amount of sleep you need declines with age with newborn babies needing as much as 18 hours compared to 6 hours for an 80 year old.

2   **Family sleeping history** – If you are from a family of short sleepers (e.g. <6 hours), it could be futile trying to achieve more than this.

3   **Recent sleep history** – If you became an insomniac in the

last 1-2 years and had a strong and regular sleeping pattern before that, use how you slept then as your guide.

4   Avoid exaggeration – There can be a large difference between how much sleep you think you need and how much your body actually needs. When you are sleep deprived it is easy to over estimate how much sleep you need in an 'eyes bigger than your stomach' kind of way. Don't expect to be able to sleep for 8 hours, having only ever slept for 6 hours when you were a normal sleeper. Trying to sleep for more hours than you need, will weaken the sleep that you do get. So for instance, 6-8 hours of good sleep is far better than 9-10 hours of fragmented poor sleep.

5   Gentle sleep restriction – A small amount of sleep restriction can be helpful for you are looking to add a little more drive into your sleep without becoming overly anxious about the fact that you now have less time in bed. Marked benefits can result from going to bed as little as 30 minutes later and getting up the same amount of time earlier for just a few weeks. You lose that extra bit of time spent lying in bed awake and so sleep more deeply and have more energy for the next day. Following such restriction for a few weeks can help to establish your new sleeping pattern.

Take a moment now to consider how many hours of sleep you need based on what you have learnt. Use this number to set the number of hours you plan to spend in bed from now on. Whatever the number, use the time to practice all that you have learnt so far and gently retrain your brain to sleep.

(*For more detailed help with sleep restriction see The Sleep School website – www.thesleepschool.org).

Quick reminders

Instant sleep – Choosing the amount of time that you plan to spend in bed does not mean that you will instantly sleep for that long. What it does do is provide the strong foundations from which your new sleeping pattern can slowly emerge and the opportunity to behave like a normal sleeper, as discussed below.

Regular pattern – Once you have chosen your new sleep duration stick with it as much as possible as this will help to strengthen the quality of your sleep in the long term. A small variation will not hurt (e.g. ±20 – 30 minutes), but try to avoid longer.

Keeping it flexible – As you get used to your new sleeping pattern you may need to fine-tune your sleep duration. Being flexible ensures that you end up with a long lasting sleeping pattern that is right for you. This could involve either restricting or adding to your sleep duration every now and then. With each change you make ensure that you leave a couple of weeks for it to take affect before changing again. Avoid changing it too often as this will lead to confusion and worsen your sleep.

Willingness – If you follow the guidelines above it is likely that the time you spend in bed is less than before so it will require willingness on your part in order to stick with it. It will mean going to bed that little bit later or getting up that little bit earlier and your mind will give you all sorts of reasons why not to do it. Watch and welcome them and carry on with the plan.

Sleep diary – If you are unsure how much time you actually spend in bed then it might be worth keeping a sleep diary for a week. This will allow you to assess whether the number of hours you spend in bed aligns with your natural sleep need and whether any changes are required. For example, you might be spending too long in bed and so it might be worth shortening the number of hours.

It will come as no surprise to you that the longer you have been awake the more sleepy you feel at night. This so called 'sleep drive' is regulated by a sleep homeostat in your brain and explains why a normal sleeper needs to be awake for at least 16 – 17 hours during the day (e.g. 7 a.m. till 11 p.m.) in order to be able to create enough drive to achieve 7 to 8 hours of sleep at night (e.g. 11 p.m. till 7 a.m.). Much like a wave on the ocean grows in size and strength, only to then break and disappear as it reaches the shore, your sleep drive rises through the day, peaking at the point of going to sleep, only to then flatten off until morning when it starts to rise all over again.

While catching this wave should be an effortless process, it can be easily missed or disturbed. For example, sleeping at the wrong times such as for too long in the morning, catching up for long periods during the day or even sleeping on the sofa while watching TV in the evening will all reduce your night time drive to sleep and so delay sleep onset. This commonly leads to feelings of frustration and anxiety about not falling to sleep, which then activate the fight or flight response, waking you up even more.

You may also suffer from 'catch up' sleep where you have a number of poor sleepless nights followed by one long blissful solid sleep. The long sleep may feel great, but if it's too long it can lead to insufficient drive for the next night and so the process is repeated. This 'catch up' sleeping can also be seen with normal sleepers who lie in on the weekend to make up for the loss during the week. When Sunday night comes even normal sleepers can lack the sleep drive required to get them to sleep. When coupled with the worries about the week ahead, it explains why Sunday is often reported as the worst night's sleep of the week.

Case Study Continued . . . John explained that the only way he could guarantee 6 hours' sleep at night, albeit broken, was if he spent at least 12 hours in bed. He achieved this by going to bed at 9 p.m. and lying in till 9 a.m. He said that it took him two hours to fall to sleep and then he would wake up every hour and a half after that for a further hour each time. He said that he resented his sleeping pattern because it affected his relationships with his wife, family and friends, but he felt helpless as to what else to do.

During the session I explained to John that his actions were very common and that while they helped him to achieve some sleep, they were inadvertently weakening his sleep drive. He realised that if he was going to improve his sleep, he would have to reduce the amount of time he spent in bed, although he described feeling very anxious at the thought of it. I suggested to him that this was very normal and that it made no sense to start restricting his sleep straight away if it was only going to further elevate his anxiety levels and therefore sleeplessness. Instead we decided to work on welcoming his anxiety and within a few weeks he was ready.

We decided on a sleep duration of eight hours, the national average. This was based on the fact that as a teenager he would sleep for 10 to 11 hours and so, given the fact that he was now in his forties, his requirement would be less. His brother and sister also now regularly slept for eight hours a night and so it was estimated it would be the correct sleep duration for him too.

When it came to his sleep timing, he decided on 11 p.m. to 7 a.m. He chose 11 p.m. as it was actually the time he naturally fell to sleep most nights. This meant he would be getting up at 7 a.m., which he liked as it would enable him to do some exercise before work, something he had not been able to do in a long time.

He described the first week as being hard because, as expected, lots of unwanted thoughts and sensations showed up, not to mention the urge to get out of bed. However, rather than being led by such thoughts and urges, he welcomed them and carried on with the plan. After a month of following his new timing, he reported that he was now falling to sleep within 30 minutes, something that he had not done for years!

When Should I Sleep?

Your body clock is a creature of habit, which explains why continually changing your sleep timing can amplify your poor sleep further. For insomniacs, the most common cause of body-clock disruption is going to bed and getting up at irregular times, or sleeping for long periods during the day. Lying in past your normal rise time resets your body clock to a new time and upsets the cycle for the next night. This further explains why Sunday nights can be problematic for so many, because the timing of your internal clock has been delayed to a later time.

The ability of your eyes to detect the changes in light levels is the primary mechanism used to keep your body clock on time. This means that as it gets dark, your brain is instructed to release the sleep-promoting hormone melatonin, which leads you to feel sleepy. In contrast, when the sun rises, the increase in light causes your melatonin production to be inhibited and your wake-promoting hormone, cortisol, to be increased, preparing you for the day ahead.

Since light acts to reset your internal clock to the correct time, it can be used to naturally overcome certain sleep disorders. For example, getting natural light onto your skin by going for a 30-minute walk outside in the morning can be a helpful way to keep your clock on time and so improve the quality of your nocturnal sleep if you suffer from insomnia. It can also be helpful to reset your clock after a bout of shift work or when recovering from jet lag.

The time of day that you receive the light can also be imporant, with the morning being ideal if you struggle to get up and the evening being better if you struggle to stay awake. The use of light-therapy boxes, which mimic the sun's rays, can also be helpful during the winter months, or if getting outside is not an option.

Choosing Your Sleep Timing

Now you know how long to sleep for, try to get some routine into when you sleep:

Keep it regular. Choose a sleep time that you can stick to, including the weekends. The more you can repeat the same regular sleeping message, the more engrained your body clock will become.

Keep it flexible. Keep your timing flexible by allowing a small amount of variation around your set times (e.g. plus or minus 30 minutes). This may seem at odds with the previous piece of advice, but having a buffer zone is exactly what normal sleepers do. If you are inflexible, you run the risk of heightening frustration and anxiety about sleep, leading to further wakefulness. Such flexibility also includes having the occasional early or late night to catch an early flight or go out with friends.

Make it workable with the rest of your life. For example, setting a rise time of 8 a.m. will not work if you have to be up earlier to get your children ready for school. It all sounds fairly obvious stuff, but when you are sleep-deprived, it's easy to create unrealistic sleeping patterns.

Listen to your body. The timing of your sleep is affected by your genetics, meaning you may be a night owl or a lark. Tune in to this because there is no point trying to go to bed at 10 p.m. if you have always naturally felt sleepy at midnight.

Get up on time. If you do have a late night after a night out, you can prevent your body clock from becoming confused by getting up at the same time as usual. This may sound like the craziest thing you have ever heard, but it prevents the time of your body clock from shifting forward, so you'll be more likely to sleep the following night. If mornings are a struggle, have a plan, as this will take the sting out of it. Set alarms, jump straight into the shower, have your clothes laid out ready and your breakfast prepared.

How Do I Become a Normal Sleeper?

When I say good sleepers do nothing, what I mean is that they don't consciously control their sleep. You can't control your sleep or the fact that your brain has learnt to keep you awake at night or fill you with fear at the thought of not sleeping. However, what you can control is how you behave in relation to not sleeping and therefore determine your sleep in the future. If you want to be a normal sleeper, then you need to start behaving like one.

Normal sleepers go about their life in a helpfully unintentional sleep-promoting way. The summation of such daily actions is that, by way of not trying to get to sleep, they do sleep.

To guide you through this process, I have broken the 24-hour period into five distinct sections entitled 'Evening', 'Wind-Down', 'Night-Time', 'Wind-Up' and 'Daytime' and will teach you the actions of normal sleepers during each of these stages, which all helpfully move them towards sleep. Normal sleepers wind down as part of the natural slowing-down process that happens every night. You too can learn simple ways in which to gradually slow down in the evening and wind down before bed. Once in bed, you can learn how to stay in a state of quiet wakefulness, saving your valuable energy for the day ahead and helpfully promoting your brain's association that the night-time is about sleepiness and rest. I will also teach you how to sleep next to your partner and let go of any of the fears that commonly surround bed-sharing. And finally you will learn how to wind up in the morning in a way that informs your brain that the day has started and defuse any unwanted struggle, enabling you to go about your day and survive feelings of extreme tiredness.

Evening

Your evening is from about 5 p.m. up to when you decide to start winding down for bed. It is traditionally considered a time for 'resting and digesting' after a long day of work and so acts as a precursor to sleep. Before street-lighting, people had no choice but to slow down during this time and so were more in tune with the natural cycle of light and dark. The benefit of this pattern is that the brain learns to associate the evening with slowing down, resting and eventually sleeping.

With the availability of artificial light, we have the capability to maintain a daytime level of activity long into the night. The result is that rest and sleepiness now have to compete for your attention against other more stimulating activities and so the message has changed, or at least become confused.

For many of us, the distinction between daytime and evening activity levels has become blurred, often at the cost of sleep. The problem is that it is easy to remain switched on as work commitments, TV, Facebook or Internet-searching all keep your brain awake. The challenge that you face is therefore learning how to adopt an evening routine that allows you to do all of these things (i.e. live your life) and yet have time to switch off properly and make sleep a priority.

What Normal Sleepers Do In the Evening

Ideally you want to achieve a gradual decline in the level of stimulation your brain and body receive over this period in preparation for your final wind-down before bed. One way to do this is to set rough time boundaries. For example, at 5 p.m. you might return home from work, pick up the kids from school or do some exercise. At 7 p.m. you might eat dinner. Then you might plan to do house chores, put the children to bed or tend to unfinished work and personal commitments for an hour or so. And finally at 9 p.m. you schedule in some recreation time, such as a chat with your partner, watch TV or listen to the radio, read, browse the Internet and so on.

There is nothing special or sleep-promoting about this routine and this is the key. You know normal sleepers do nothing to sleep other than behave in a way that moves them gently towards sleep, rather than away. Establishing a pattern can be a helpful way to promote improved sleep as your brain begins to reassociate the evening period with switching off. Having said this, it is important to keep such time boundaries flexible and workable with the rest of your life. There will of course always be times when you can't follow such a routine because you decide to go out with friends and so be it. Starting to behave in this flexible and relaxed manner is the key to becoming a normal sleeper once more.

And of course once you start sleeping more normally, you'll forget you even have a wind-down pattern. It will just happen naturally.

Wind-Down

Your wind-down involves everything you do 30 to 45 minutes before going to bed and turning out the light. The idea is to further lower your energy, alertness, activity and light levels from that of the evening phase.

The aim of this time period is for you to be relaxed and so it makes sense for you to avoid any excessive stimulation. If you keep up a daytime level of activity and light stimulation right up to the point of going to sleep on a regular basis, you are reducing your brain's ability to switch off at night. This is why most traditional sleep therapists impose rules, such as the bedroom is for sleep and sex only. The reasoning being that this will stop any unwanted stimulating activity and so increase the likelihood of falling to sleep.

While such rules can create a non-stimulating environment, they lack long-term workability because normal sleepers do not follow them. The main emphasis of the Sleep School approach is to let go of the effort involved in preparing yourself to sleep. Only by freeing yourself from the rules and rituals can you get back to a normal wind-down.

What Normal Sleepers Do to Wind Down

The three simple steps typically performed by a normal sleeper during their wind-down are:

- Stop all stimulating activities 30 to 45 minutes before going to bed, such as watching TV, listening to the radio or music, emailing, phoning, texting and playing computer games, if you have not already done so.
- Engage in gentle end-of-day activities such as having a warm drink, getting ready for the next day, locking doors, brushing teeth and changing into nightwear.
- Get into bed and read a book or magazine, chat with your partner and then turn out the light in preparation for sleep.

Like the evening phase, this wind-down is not performed with the intention of promoting sleep, rather it respects the brain's need to be told that sleep is on its way. You should do this at roughly the same time most nights.

In this way it could be described as a sort of ritual, although one that you are not reliant on in order to sleep. All of the actions are performed out of habit (e.g. locking the doors), enjoyment (e.g. having a warm drink) or as part of a natural transition towards your bed (e.g. getting undressed).

It is flexible, so if you want to watch a movie with your family every once in a while, you can. In this instance it is ok to leave everything till the morning and get quickly into bed and turn out the lights. The paradox is that by not trying to adopt a sleep-focused wind-down, you naturally take the pressure off yourself to sleep and therefore increase the chance of actually sleeping.

SLEEP FACT

A hypnic jerk is the feeling of falling that occurs as you start to sleep and results in a sudden waking jolt in your arms and legs. It is believed to occur because the brain misinterprets the natural relaxation of the muscles upon falling to sleep as the body actually falling and so jolts you awake to regain balance. Almost everyone will experience them during their lifetime and they are completely harmless, though a little annoying.

Unfortunately, their frequency tends to increase with tiredness and so for many of my clients, it can feel like they are stuck in a vicious cycle whereby they finally manage to fall off to sleep only to have their body jolt them awake again. While it can be challenging to not get annoyed or be fearful of these jolts, the key is to mindfully acknowledge them and carry on with being in bed. The more playful you can be, the better, such as saying, 'Here are my little jerks again,' each time they happen.

Another distressing occurrence that many clients report as they fall to sleep is a sudden surge of adrenaline through their body that jolts them awake. Many describe it like a bolt of lightning that leaves them wired, anxious, hyper-alert and with their heart racing. It is believed to occur because the brain now associates failing to sleep with danger and so releases stress hormones to prepare you to stand and fight or run away in flight. For many clients, it becomes a further source of sleep anxiety and is therefore self-perpetuating. Once again responding to it in a gently playful manner, such as saying, 'Here is the bolt,' and then mindfully returning your attention to your bed is the best way to signal to the brain that no threat exists and that it is okay for sleep to emerge.

Night-Time

This is the time between when you turn out the light at the end of your wind-down to when you get out of bed in the morning at the start of your wind-up.

What Normal Sleepers Do at Night

When the lights go out at the start of the night, a normal sleeper will close their eyes, make themselves comfortable and then lie quietly until they fall asleep. This pre-sleep phase involves a waxing and waning of consciousness levels as the brain moves between wakefulness and light sleep. During this time the mind gently ponders over the events of the day or flashes up a collection of images or memories from your life so far. It can flit easily between internal thoughts about yourself or external thoughts about the world around you, with no obvious agenda.

Falling asleep is therefore a gradual process of disengagement over time, rather than a sudden turning-off of a switch. This explains why most people when tested in sleep laboratories and woken from light sleep will report that they have been awake when actually they were asleep. Technically the brain is in the first light stage of sleep, as measured by its electrical activity, but our conscious awareness of the outside world is such that what we can hear and feel remains turned on for several minutes until we fall into deep sleep.

The most important thing to note about a normal sleeper is their willingness to relax and be quietly wakeful in the pre-sleep phase. They aren't trying to force sleep upon themselves, but are happy to ride along with it, knowing that even if they don't sleep, they are still getting some much-needed rest.

You may have read the above sentences and either thought that it sounds fantastic or impossible or both! You may feel a long way off from this place right now, but this feeling won't last. Following this programme will help you to behave in a way that allows you to relax in the pre-sleep phase, save your energy and ultimately become a normal sleeper.

The Olympic Podium of Night-Time Activity

This is a highly effective concept I use at the Sleep School. The three medal positions depicted in the illustration highlight the potential outcome of different ways of behaving at night. Your actions will determine where you currently sit in the medal table.

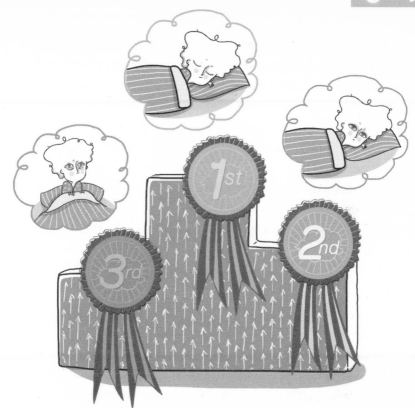

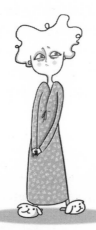

Fig. 4.2 **The Medals Podium of Sleep**

Gold medal

The gold medal goes to you when you are lying in bed asleep, as this is when you conserve the most energy and get rest. If you are in a relationship, this position also sees you being able to share a bed with your partner.

Silver medal

The silver medal is given when you are lying in bed with your eyes closed in a state of quiet wakefulness, while waiting for sleep to come. When you are able to do this, you are in the pre-sleep phase, and if you can be calm in this place, you'll be well on your way to working up to the gold-medal position.

Here you accept the fact that you are awake and are willing to 'watch' and 'welcome' any of your wanted or unwanted thoughts, memories, images or sensations that arise in your mind and body moment by moment. You take the position of a peaceful bystander who watches over your internal world without judgement or comment.

In this position you mindfully focus your energy on the benefits of being in bed and resting. Rest is an insomniac's lifeline as it saves your valuable energy for the day ahead so that you can start living your life once more. You recognise that paradoxically the key to sleeping is having an accepting and relaxed attitude towards being awake at night. When you can let go of the idea that you need to be asleep, then you remove the obstacles in the way of falling to sleep.

Being in this phase does not instantly mean that you sleep, but repeatedly responding in this helpful way confirms to your brain that the night-time is about sleepiness and rest. Over time this makes space for natural sleep to emerge.

Crucially it undoes any unhelpful sleep associations that have formed from previous nights of struggle and starts a new chapter in your sleeping life.

Bronze medal

The bronze medal also goes to lying in bed awake, except in this state there's less acceptance and more struggle, anxiety, frustration and resignation. Here your unwillingness to experience wakefulness or any of the thoughts and sensations that present themselves begins to amplify your insomnia. When you use unhelpful coping strategies to get yourself to sleep, you inadvertently increase your level of brain stimulation, which pushes you further away from the pre-sleep phase.

In this state and in the no-medals position it's common to avoid bed-sharing by sleeping in the spare room or on the couch in an attempt to control your sleeping environment. If allowed to continue, such actions reinforce your brain's unhelpful association that the night-time is about wakefulness and struggle and so wake you up again night after night.

No medals

This position refers to getting out of bed in the night-time and engaging in activities to avoid being with the wakefulness, thoughts and sensations associated with not sleeping. This position sees the lowest level of energy conservation and greatest level of stimulation, and the fact that you are no longer in your bed means you are the furthest away from sleep.

Moving Up the Medals Podium

Most people starting this programme are in the no-medals or bronze position, but soon learn how to steadily move into the silver- and then gold-medal positions. By now you have a good idea of where you sit in the medal table and can see where you'd like to go next, but the key is your willingness to move up. Outlined below are some of the common barriers to moving up that podium, along with some helpful advice on how to get around them.

Being awake in bed

It helps enormously to view night-time wakefulness as an opportunity to gently get to know your insomnia. If you can do this, try to use it as time to be still and rest, and to put into practice all of the tools that you have learnt so far. If you have forgotten how to mindfully 'watch' your insomnia, then revisit 'Exercise: Noticing at Night' as discussed in Week 2. Remember that watching is neither a way of forcing yourself to sleep or distracting yourself from the fact that you are not sleeping. Instead it is a gentle level of wakeful awareness that prepares you for being in the pre-sleep phase.

One of the immediate differences to be seen by being willing to be awake in bed is the amount of energy you have the next day. In spite of not actually sleeping any better at first, many patients report that the absence of night-time struggle and focus on rest means that they have more daytime energy. This can have a powerful effect because the more clients start to resume their daytime lives, the less they struggle with sleep at night, helping them to escape the vicious cycle of insomnia as depicted in Week 1.

Staying in bed

If you have habitually escaped the bedroom in the middle of the night as a way of coping with your insomnia, choosing to stay in bed can feel like the worst thing in the world. If this is the case for you, then it can be helpful to gradually build up to it because there is no point in lying in bed rigid with fear and anxiety. Remember, the aim is to gently increase your willingness to experience quiet wakefulness so that you can effortlessly access the pre-sleep phase like a normal sleeper.

A halfway house you can use if you need a short break is to sit on the edge of the bed for a few minutes. It can create a little bit of separation between you and the bed, as well as a sense of perspective on whatever discomfort has arrived, before returning under the covers. You can use this as an opportunity to practise your mindfulness exercises to enable you to achieve that objectivity and let go of the judgement. If repeated, this practice can help you to break the cycle of needing to get out of bed altogether and so move you further up the medal podium. If you feel that you really need to leave the bedroom, then do so, but keep it short and non-stimulating.

At the start it can be helpful to have a plan for how long each night you are willing to stay in bed with your insomnia before getting out for a break. Aim to gradually reduce the amount of time spent out of bed and the frequency of trips per night. Clients who have followed this approach have found that they can quite quickly increase the amount of time they spend in bed and notice improvements in their energy levels as a result.

Please note that staying in bed does not include your need to go to the toilet, which is perfectly natural once per night. However, if, like some of my clients, your bedroom avoidance is based around continuously going to the toilet, then this habit needs to be curbed as well.

Many traditional sleep therapists use a technique known as the 'Quarter Hour Rule' to deal with insomnia. The aim of this is to reduce the amount of time you could possibly lie in bed struggling with sleep and so limit the opportunity for any unhelpful association with sleep to be formed. It requires individuals to get out of bed if they have been awake for more than 15 minutes and go to a spare room and do something quiet and relaxing such as read a boring book. The hope is that by getting out of bed and distracting yourself, it will help to calm any unwanted anxieties and increase your sleepiness levels so that when you return to bed, you fall quickly to sleep.

While this technique does work for some people, it is questionable as to whether escaping the bedroom is the most effective way to go about building a helpful long-term relationship with your sleep. If the aim is to limit the amount you struggle, then surely the focus should be on why you do it in the first place, rather than how you can avoid it. It solves the problem in the short term, but is not a long-term workable solution to overcoming your fear.

In some individuals who have tried this 'getting up' approach, it can be seen that they have unhelpfully created a new association that the night-time is about getting up and being active. In many of these cases, the act of escaping the bed is often used as a way of avoiding the discomfort that comes with insomnia. If this is the case, many clients report their unwanted thoughts and feelings waiting for them when they return to bed and thus feel helpless as to what to do with them, other than simply escape again.

Another commonly reported problem that I see with this technique is in its implementation with clients who would rather stay in their beds. For them, being forced out because they are awake feels most unintuitive and can actually increase anxiety levels and so push sleep further away.

Normal sleepers do not get out of bed if they can't sleep and neither should you. The aim is to help you to be willing to be in bed with all of your fears rather than running around the house doing things to avoid them. I firmly believe that the most workable way of building a helpful relationship with your sleep is therefore by gradually learning how to be in bed with your fears, rather than out of bed escaping them. Once you are happy to be in bed awake, you are already closer to sleep, but with the added benefit of saving your valuable energy for the next day.

Case Study Continued . . . Another issue for John was his habit of getting out of bed if he woke and going downstairs and doing something boring. He'd been told to do this by another sleep specialist and continued with it because it helped to lessen his night-time anxiety and overcame the boredom of just lying awake in bed all night. Unfortunately, it had not improved his sleep, and if anything, he felt like his body had got into the habit of waking him up to do stuff! I explained that while getting out of bed can help people to relieve their unwanted emotions in the short term, in the long term it can actually perpetuate wakefulness. Learning to welcome his anxiety in the middle of the night changed everything because he no longer felt he needed to get up and distract himself. Instead he could now enjoy the comfort of his bed and benefit from the rest he was getting from just lying still. Plus because he no longer feared staying in bed, he soon found that he typically fell back to sleep minutes after he had woken.

Clock-watching

Constantly checking the time and calculating how much time you have left to sleep is a common problem of being awake in bed. An easy way to solve the problem is to remove the clock from view to prevent any unwanted checking and further anxiety. However, since the problem lies in your reaction to the time, rather than with the clock itself, simply avoiding it is not a long-term solution, although it can be a helpful first step. The key is to change your relationship with the time. For example, if a normal sleeper wakes up at 3 a.m. and looks at the clock, knowing that they have to be up at 6 a.m. for work, they will be pleased that they have three more hours in bed and normally fall back to sleep. In contrast, if an insomniac wakes up in the same situation, they will often spend their time worrying about how they only have three hours left before they have to get up, and so stay awake. Once you are able to notice and let go of worrying thoughts and are willing to experience unwanted emotions as shown in Weeks 2 and 3, you'll let go of the need to constantly check the clock.

Sharing your bed

Most sleep therapists suggest moving into a separate room. I stongly disagree with this as sharing a bed brings a sense of love, comfort and even safety to the bedroom; unfortunately, it also comes with an increased level of sleep disturbance in the form of unwanted noise, movement and differing bed-times and temperature requirements. Such disturbance can be the source of much bedroom anxiety and sleeplessness, with clients either worrying about how much their partner will disturb their sleep or how much they will disturb their partner's sleep with their constant tossing and turning throughout the night. For some clients, the fear of bed-sharing is so strong that it has disuaded them from ever entering into a relationship!

For your thinking mind, the obvious solution to this bed-sharing issue is easy and typically involves yourself or your partner moving out of the main bedroom to sleep on the couch or in the spare room. In the short term this can supply you with an increased sense of control over your environment and possibly result in an improvement in sleep. However, if such activity becomes habit, it can potentially increase the fear surrounding bed-sharing and promote further poor sleep in the long term. For many of my clients, it also goes against a basic value of wanting to be able to share a bed with someone they love, which explains why much of my time is spent teaching clients how to share a bed again.

If you have spent many years sleeping apart from your partner, the thought of sleeping in the same bed again can be daunting. More than likely many of your unhelpful thoughts and sensations will want to join in on the experience (as discussed in Week 3). Once again your willingness to share your bed with those unwanted arrivals will determine whether you stay in bed with your partner or escape to the spare room.

You can do this slowly over a number of weeks by gradually increasing the amount of nights spent sharing a bed. If the thought of spending a whole night bed-sharing is too much, then you might want to start with 30 minutes or an hour per night and then build up from there.

By using all of the mindfulness and welcoming techniques discussed in Weeks 2 and 3, the aim is to gently increase your willingness to experience all of the thoughts, emotions and sensations that show up and begin to realise that despite not being very nice, they cannot harm you.

You many think now isn't the right time because of work and life commitments. There will be better times than others, but there is never a perfect time and waiting for one can simply delay the inevitable. Choose a start date and run with it, and be flexible enough to adapt to any life events that may arise along the way.

If you struggle to sleep on your own, then you may feel inclined to work on this area before tackling the issue of sharing a bed. This can appear to be the most effective approach, as it lessens the amount that you have to deal with all at once. However, it can also result in clients learning to sleep well on their own, but then never making the final step to bed-sharing because they are unwilling to go back to sleeping badly again. It often makes sense to tackle this issue at the same time as learning to sleep well. They involve the same techniques, so you will be better off in the long run. Involve your partner too. That way they do not feel left out of the loop and can offer much-needed support in the middle of the night.

Case Study Continued . . . John described that sleeping in the spare room was a coping mechanism for him as he no longer needed to be worried about being disturbed by his wife's snoring or movements. It also allowed him to control the wave of jealousy, anger and then loneliness that rose up inside him as a result of watching his wife fall to sleep as soon as her head hit the pillow. Unfortunately, while such actions had improved his sleep at first, over time he now slept just as badly on his own and completely feared the thought of bed-sharing again. This meant that he and his wife tended not to go away anymore unless they could guarantee separate bedrooms.

Since sharing a bed with his wife was of such value to him, we decided on a plan to achieve this. The first thing we did was note down all of the unwanted thoughts that were likely to show up when attempting to share a bed with his wife, such as 'I can't believe she is asleep already' or 'She is going to start snoring soon', and the emotional responses, such as the waves of anxiety and adrenaline that would course through his body. I emphasised the fact that while he could not stop such experiences from occurring, he could learn to respond to them in a more helpful way than simply escaping to the spare room.

Over a period of a month he then gradually started to increase the amount of time he spent sharing a bed. He described that the first few nights, when he would stay for a few hours at a time, were awful and he literally could not wait to get out of bed and go back to the safety of the spare room. However, after a couple of weeks he discovered that the symptoms no longer mattered and paled into significance when compared to the importance of sharing a bed with his wife. He used this as his motivation and after a month of practice was able to report waking up in the morning next to his wife for the first time in years.

The Wind-Up

Winding up in the morning can be as helpful to your day as your wind-down is to your night. Getting light on your skin tells your body clock to stop producing the sleep-promoting hormone melatonin and start producing the waking hormone cortisol. It is the chemical starting gun for your day, but also your brain's countdown towards your next sleep. If you struggle in the morning, having a regular wind-up plan can also be a way of defusing pent-up night-time emotion, which would otherwise be unhelpfully vented on your partner, your children or unsuspecting work colleagues.

What Normal Sleepers Do to Wind Up

In the morning normal sleepers will:

- Get up out of bed at roughly the same time most days of the week, including on the weekend.
- Open the curtains, turn on the lights, have a shower, turn on the radio or TV.
- Eat a healthy breakfast, have a cup of coffee or tea, do some exercise, get the kids ready for school, go to work and so on.

The wind-up routine is common sense and what most normal sleepers just do. The problem is that when you have not slept, it is easy to get out of your normal rhythm. Many insomniacs abandon a gentle wind-up in favour of staying in bed till the very last minute, then rushing to work with no breakfast. Unfortunately, starting the day in this chaotic way sets off another vicious cycle with the wrong tone for the day ahead and then the night to come.

Find your own regular morning rhythm that fits in with the rest of your life. If on the weekend you want to lie in bed awake with your partner, read the newspapers, have breakfast or even play with your children, then do it, as it helps to cultivate a good relationship with your bed.

As your trust in your natural ability to sleep improves, then you can even start to be a little more flexible with your wake-up time. For example, lying in for an extra hour on the weekend every once in a while will not disturb your sleep-wake cycle. Problems only arise if the morning becomes a time when you repeatedly catch up on your sleep, as discussed earlier.

Daytime

Being awake in the daytime builds up your natural drive to sleep. However, as an insomniac, daytime tiredness can be a major challenge. Here you'll find some extra practical approaches that can help you stay awake during the day and yet promote sleep at night.

What Normal Sleepers Do In the Daytime

One way in which many normal sleepers tackle daytime tiredness is to take a short nap in the middle of the day as a way of recharging themselves and still sleep well at night. Much like an over-tired baby will not be able to sleep, a 'tired but wired' insomniac can't either, so taking a short nap has the capacity to lessen excessive tiredness, defuse unwanted anxiety and slow the racing mind in preparation for the night ahead.

Exercise: The Normal Sleeper's Three-Step Nap

If you practise this, then we really believe you'll eventually find that sleep will come quickly.

○ Choose a time, ideally after lunch or in the early afternoon, to take a short 10- to 20-minute nap. Avoid napping past 3 p.m.

○ Find a quiet, dark and comfortable place to sit or lie down where you will not be disturbed.

○ Close your eyes and allow yourself to enter the pre-sleep phase of quiet wakefulness. If your mind won't stop racing, then use the time to do your mindful breathing practice. If you feel you might sleep too long, then set an alarm.

○ If you're pretty sure you won't actually sleep, don't worry. Take sleep out of the equation and view it as an opportunity to practise being in a state of quiet wakefulness. The focus is on gaining valuable rest rather than trying to sleep.

The key is to nap for no more than 20 minutes, as this prevents you from excessively weakening your sleep drive if you do actually fall to sleep. It also prevents you experiencing brain fog, which happens when you wake yourself from deep sleep.

If you're pregnant, have just had a baby or have any serious health issues, you'll have extra demands on your energy levels, so do nap for longer: you could have a whole 90-minute sleep cycle. It's important for you to get through whatever additional stress you are experiencing and then start to work on creating a robust sleep-wake cycle once your health has returned.

Being active and living

When you are feeling really tired in the day, the urge to roll up into a ball and escape from the world can sometimes be overwhelming. Retreating like this can be helpful, especially if you are feeling ill or coming down with a cold.

At other times it can be helpful to be active and to get on with living your life with your tiredness. You can get a huge boost from going for a 20-minute walk at lunchtime as a way of making it through the day. The natural light stimulates your wakefulness levels, and the gentle exercise releases endorphins, helping to boost your mood. You don't need to run a marathon to do this, but just gently inform your brain that you are willing to carry on with your life, no matter how small the action may be.

Helpful Sleep Habits

Most of the activities so far have been to learn to let go of struggling with the things that you can't change, such as your thoughts, emotional responses and your sleeplessness. However, it is also helpful to change the things that can be changed if they move you closer towards natural sleep.

This section is therefore focused on the changes that you can make to your lifestyle that will have a helpful effect on your sleep.

Sleep Hygiene

'Sleep hygiene' is the term given to controlling all aspects of your environment and lifestyle that could potentially interfere with the quality of your sleep. This is covered extensively in traditional sleep advice, so I will just touch on it here and you can find more information on the Sleep School website.

Research shows that your sleep is improved if your bedroom is cool, clean, comfortable, quiet and dark. Living a healthy lifestyle is also shown to be helpful, which explains why such information is routinely handed out at every doctor's surgery. It includes sensible advice such as ensuring that you sleep in a darkened room, get lots of exercise and drink less stimulants such as caffeine. However, if you are anything like the majority of insomniacs, you may well have done all of this and still not slept. I often joke with clients that they probably have the best bedrooms in the world or that they are the healthiest people I know, simply because of all the changes they have made in order to get a good night's sleep.

If you haven't yet made changes in this way, then relax – you may not have to. They don't guarantee improved sleep and, if obsessed over, can become part of the problem. The key lies in doing what is helpful for your sleep, and by this I mean making changes to your bedroom and lifestyle only when and where they are needed. All of the information here is designed to give you a balanced view of many of the helpful sleep habits that are often discussed and where to draw the line in the level of attention you give them.

Bedroom Environment
Light
Light plays an important role in the regulation of your sleep-wake cycle and we sleep best in darkened conditions. While the room does not need to be pitch black, it can be helpful to have a good set of curtains, blinds or use an eye mask, especially in the summer months. Getting rid of unnecessary

artificial lights such LED clocks or any other standby lights will also help.

Temperature

We sleep best in cool environments, ideally around 17–19 degrees Celsius (63–66 degrees Fahrenheit). When temperatures go above or below that, your body can become restless and your sleep disturbed.

If you feel excessively hot, sweaty or experience hot flushes in the night, remember it's how you react that determines how much it affects your ability to sleep. Choosing to struggle with it by constantly tossing and turning, huffing and puffing, flinging the covers off and on or getting in and out of bed will only exacerbate the situation. Choosing to objectively watch and welcome the sensations of heat in your body and the unhelpful thoughts in your mind won't make them go away, but won't amplify them either.

SLEEP FACT ☾

Your body has millions of sensors both inside and out that are continually sending data to your brain about your current situation. Your eyes and ears give you the power to see and hear things in your environment. Touch and temperature sensors in your skin help you to detect the feel of your clothes or whether you are hot or cold. Stretch and pain receptors in your muscles give you feedback about your position and level of pain.

All of this information is fed into the waking centre part of your brain known as your reticular activating system. If a high level of information is being received, then it is likely that you will have an accordingly high

> level of alertness or wakefulness. This explains the
> benefits of closing your eyes and being in a dark, quiet,
> cool and comfortable room when attempting to sleep
> because it helps to minimise the amount of sensory
> information that your brain receives and so push you
> closer to sleep.

Beds and mattresses

Without becoming obsessed, just be aware that the comfort
of your bed can play a role in the quality of your sleep, especially if you share a bed. Having enough space to move around
can reduce the chance of being woken by your partner.

Your choice of bedding and pillow can also affect the quality
of your sleep, just like your mattress. Ultimately the choice is
yours and experimentation is the key.

Equally, what you wear in bed can affect your level of
comfort and therefore your sleep quality. Aim for loose-fitting
and comfortable nightwear that allow for easy movement
and breathability.

There are some helpful tips on our website if you need
more detailed advice.

Noise

Noise can be the bane of your life if you have insomnia: it can
both trigger and maintain sleeplessness. During the lighter
phases of sleep it may only require someone gently opening a
door or footsteps across a room for your sleep to be disturbed.
This means that snoring partners, partying neighbours, crying
babies, barking dogs, beeping cars, planes taking off or even
nice sounds like the dawn chorus can all disturb your sleep.
One simple way of controlling this is to use earplugs.

A couple of things to be aware of, however. Firstly, while they block out all external noise, the newfound silence makes you more aware of internal noises that can keep you awake, such as the beating of your heart. And secondly, don't let them become a prop that you become reliant on in order to sleep. It is vital that you use them only when they are actually needed. If you would like to know what environmental sleep products and brands I recommend, then please visit www.thesleep-school.org.

Lifestyle Habits
Caffeine

Caffeine is one of the first things to be cut out whenever someone starts to experience insomnia, but I don't necessarily agree with this, unless you are super sensitive to caffeine, in which case it makes no sense to drink it when you have insomnia.

The key is balance and finding a level of consumption that is both workable for your life and your sleep. If you cut it out completely, you run the risk of it becoming yet another thing that you do to solve your insomnia, something that can place sleep further on a pedestal, raise anxiety levels and push your goal further away. Equally, if you are consuming lots as a way of coping with the tiredness that comes with poor sleep, then it is likely to affect the quality of any sleep that you do actually achieve. It's probably wise to have no more than two or three cups in total and knock it on the head by early afternoon (i.e. just after lunch). If you fancy a warm drink at a later stage, then opt for one of the many herbal teas available or try decaf, although beware that this still does contain a small amount of caffeine.

Adenosine is a substance that builds up in the brain during every hour that you are awake and is thought to contribute to the natural increase in your sleep drive that occurs at the same time. Its action is to slow down your nervous system and so it makes sense that it could be responsible for feelings of drowsiness and sleepiness that occur as the day goes on.

Caffeine is the antagonist of adenosine, which means that it blocks the use of adenosine by the brain. This explains why your nervous system speeds up after you have a coffee or a tea. Drinking too much caffeine or drinking it too late can potentially diminish your sleep drive and push you further away from sleep.

Alcohol

Having the odd glass of wine with an evening meal can be an enjoyable thing to do. However, when it comes to improving your sleep, this is often one of the first things to go and so yet another example of 'trying' to make yourself sleep and a possible source of sleep anxiety. Once again, finding a balance and understanding all the facts is the key. Alcohol can make you feel more relaxed and sleepy; however, if drunk to excess and close to bedtime, it can cause shallow and disturbed sleep, abnormal dreams and frequent early morning awakenings.

It takes your body an hour to metabolise one unit of alcohol. This means that if you have a standard-sized glass of wine (i.e. 2.5 units) with a meal at 7 p.m., it will be mostly cleared from your system by 9.30 p.m. and therefore have very little effect on your sleep. If you are very sensitive to alcohol or have a slow metabolism, then this process could take longer. So go ahead and have the odd glass of wine with a meal if it is something you enjoy. Having said this, if you regularly drink more than one or two glasses a night, then the alcohol content of your bloodstream during sleep could be a problem. Cutting down could prove helpful for both your sleep and your long-term health.

It's common for my chronic insomniacs to have used alcohol to sleep or as a way of silencing a racing mind or lessening anxious feelings. While it may work to knock you out, the sleep is not restorative and you'll wake up the next day feeling tired, if not hung-over. The added health implications mean that it is not an ideal long-term coping strategy. If you feel that you now can't sleep without using alcohol, then learning to sit with the urge as discussed in Week 3 should help. If the problem remains, then discuss your situation with your GP.

Smoking

Smoking is often used as a coping strategy for stress, so insomniacs resort to it just before going to bed or in the middle of the night. While smoking may give you a sense of being calm and relaxed, nicotine is a stimulant and therefore wakes you up.

Obviously giving up would be good, but at the very least have your last cigarette four hours before going to bed and avoid all smoking in the middle of the night.

Cannabis

Smoking cannabis makes you drowsy and many people find that it helps them to relax and drift off to sleep. Research shows that while it may help you drop off to sleep, it actually appears to interfere with the later stages of sleep, fragmenting it and leaving you more tired in the morning. Smoking cannabis can also be associated with paranoia, something that does not help if your mind is already over-tired and brimming with worrisome thoughts.

Exercise

Being physically active during the day can help to break down muscle and tire out the body, two factors that can be helpful in promoting a sound night's sleep. However, it does not guarantee it and I have worked with insomniacs who have literally been running marathons to tire themselves out but have ended up lying awake all night physically shattered and yet mentally alert. As with many lifestyle habits, the key point here is your intention. If you are exercising because it is an enjoyable, healthy thing to do, then it can have a positive impact on your sleep. However, if you are doing it with the intention of getting to sleep, you run the risk of placing yet more unwanted pressure and anxiety on yourself and inadvertently pushing sleep further away.

Aim to be active every day by going out for a walk in the fresh air for at least 20 minutes. It is amazing how even a short walk can raise endorphin levels and elevate your mood, as well as being good for your physical health. If you have more time, exercise for at least 30 minutes, 3 times per week, making sure you are increasing your heart and breathing rate, as well as getting a bit sweaty. If you have a bad night and don't feel like exercising, it's often worth pushing yourself to do it, as generally you'll feel better. You don't need to push yourself super hard, though; just be active. Ideally exercising in the morning or afternoon is best. However, people's sensitivity to exercise varies, so experiment with what works for you.

Diet

Eating healthy food supplies the body with essential nutrients and energy that help with growth and repair, and promote good mental health and well-being. Most sleep advice suggests using food to help sleep on the basis that certain foods contain the sleep-promoting hormone melatonin or the amino acids tryptophan and serotonin, which can be used by the body to make melatonin. So-called 'sleepy' foods include pumpkin seeds, almonds, tofu, chicken, turkey, lettuce, sweetcorn, bananas, tomatoes, rice, potatoes and pasta. While it is true that many of these foods do contain these chemicals, they are in such small quantities that they will have very little effect on your sleep and potentially lead to yet further sleep anxiety if they don't work.

Your time and effort are better spent on avoiding certain sleep-disturbing foods close to bedtime or managing the amount you eat. For example, eating sugary snacks in the evening can lower your blood glucose and cause you to wake up hungry in the night. The same goes for eating chocolate too close to bedtime. Equally, eating a hot curry or some strong cheese before heading to bed could easily disturb your sleep. If you eat to excess at the point of going to bed, then you also run the risk of spending the night digesting your food and being awake. Eat a light healthy meal at least a couple of hours before going to bed. If you feel hungry before bedtime, then have a small snack such as natural yoghurt, a banana or a small bowl of muesli to tide you over till the morning.

One of the problems with poor sleep and tiredness is that it alters the hormones that regulate your appetite and satiety levels. This probably explains why you always feel like eating sugary foods and have the urge to eat larger portions when you are tired. Being able to sit with such urges, rather than giving in to them is therefore important.

Many of you will also wake in the middle of the night feeling hungry and so go downstairs to eat something as a way of solving the problem. While this technique does sometimes work, if you are repeatedly eating an extra meal, then you will soon put on weight. You also run the risk of your brain becoming conditioned to waking you up to eat at this time. Such behaviour can create unhelpful beliefs such as 'I can't sleep unless I have had my midnight snack', which promotes an inflexible relationship with sleep.

The night-time is a fasting time and so it is perfectly normal to feel hungry, the only point is that we are normally asleep and so don't notice it. If this is a problem for you, then the exercises in Weeks 2 and 3 will help you get to know your hunger and let go of the need to do something about it in the night.

Health
Your health plays an important role in the quality of your sleep and so doing all you can to maintain it is helpful. As discussed in Week 1, insomnia can be secondary to a number of mental and physical health conditions such as depression, anxiety, chronic pain, arthritis, cancer, cardiovascular disease, chronic fatigue, tinnitus or even another sleep disorder such as sleep apnoea or restless-leg syndrome. Getting the correct medical help and treatment for such conditions is vital for improving your sleep, while also following this plan.

LIVE
...your days to the full and sleep well every night

'But he who dares not grasp the thorn
Should never crave the rose'

Anne Brontë

This week, in the final phase of the programme, we will:

- Make plans for the rest of your life, as living your best life helps you sleep at night.
- Rejoin the world fully to live the life you want to live, rather than losing it to an endless battle with insomnia.
- Learn how to maintain good sleep by calmly dealing with insomnia if it recurs, just like a normal sleeper would.

Client Case Study: Patricia and Her Narrowed Life

Patricia began sleeping badly the moment she started working after leaving university. She described how in the three years since then she had been on a mission to find the cause of her poor sleep. She blamed her insomnia for ruining her life and described how she had helplessly watched it narrow to almost nothing.

She had given up her first job because she thought it might be the stress that was causing the problem. She ended her relationship because she could not sleep when her boyfriend was around and the more they argued, the worse her sleep became. She moved back to her parents' place because she used to be able to sleep well at home and the country was a lot quieter than living in the city. She stopped socialising with her friends at night because she worried it would affect her sleep. Plus since she was following all of the recommended guidelines about not drinking alcohol or caffeine and only eating certain foods at certain times, it made going out very challenging. She tried exhausting herself through exercise, but then stopped it altogether because it did not work and only seemed to make her feel more awake.

Instead, most of her days were now spent thinking about her sleep, and all of her waking energy, which included most nights, was focused on trying to solve the problem of why she could not sleep.

By the time she came to see me, she was exhausted mentally and physically. She was desperate, lonely, depressed and convinced that she was a lost cause and that she would never sleep properly again. She described to me how she had no life left and how insomnia had ruined everything and she felt like a freak.

During our first session I explained how all of her efforts to fix her poor sleep and make the pain go away were normal but also part of the problem. I mentioned that while she blamed her insomnia for everything that had happened, in reality it was her fear of experiencing it and then her ongoing attempts to control it that had driven her to stop living her life. I explained that the only thing getting in her way was herself and that if she was willing to face her fears, she could start to live her life and retrain her brain to sleep at the same time.

Re-live your life

Most insomniacs have restricted their lives in order to control their sleeplessness. Patricia is an extreme example, but some of her actions may have resonated with you and the way you live your life.

As your focus narrows onto fixing your insomnia you can lose sight of what is important to you or put it on hold in the hope of sleeping. Living in the service of getting rid of your insomnia is not really living because it makes you more isolated, stressed, anxious all of which helps to keep you awake.

Being desperate to try anything to sleep, life gets pushed to the back of the queue, as all your energy gets diverted into trying to get rid of the sleepless nights and the consequences. To your logical 'problem solving' brain, doing something that will alleviate your pain and suffering is worth doing.

So, if going out with friends at night means that you spend the time 'clock watching' and worrying about whether you will be able to sleep and how you will feel if you don't, then the obvious solution is to avoid going out. Equally, if sharing a bed with your partner causes you to feel overly anxious because your sleep will be disturbed by their noise and movement, then moving to the spare room where it is quiet and still, is again the obvious solution.

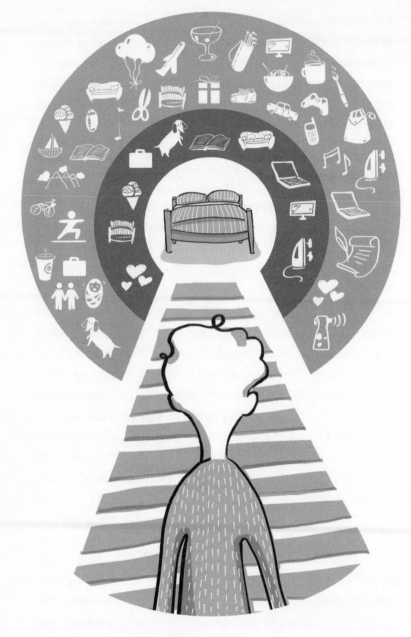

Fig. 5.1 **How Insomnia Narrows Your Life**

Whatever the scenario, when you are faced with such discomfort your thinking mind quickly comes up with ways of trying to control or avoid it.

This kind of pain avoidance is not confined to the realms of insomnia. We all have times in our lives when we've chosen not to do something to avoid the possibility of experiencing pain: deciding not to go for a job interview to avoid feeling rejected; breaking off a relationship just as it was getting serious to avoid heartbreak or giving up on a diet to avoid the pain of feeling hungry.

While avoiding such discomfort and vulnerability makes perfect sense to your logical thinking mind which is always seeking to protect you from pain and suffering in your life, the effect is short lasting.

If you are not prepared to feel rejected, anxious, heartbroken, achy or hungry, then you may never get to live the life you wish for. A life without pain and discomfort comes at the cost of your life itself. You cannot have one without the other. It is only when you open yourself up to being vulnerable and the possibility of experiencing pain that you can live.

Living your life is therefore the final stage to curing your insomnia because although you acknowledge the presence of insomnia you make the conscious choice not to let it run your life.

The paradox is that by choosing to live your life with your insomnia, rather than in spite of it, you take away the reason for struggling with sleeplessness in the first place. Less struggle means less night-time arousal, less wasted energy and therefore more capacity for living a rich and meaningful life, something that creates an environment from which natural sleep can emerge.

We struggle against insomnia because our mind fears the consequences of not sleeping and imagines how much it will affect the rest of our life. The problem is our response. Giving up part or all of your life in order to control your insomnia, so that you can get back to living your life is not a workable equation but just another vicious circle.

In order to sleep well you have added in the additional problem of not living your life, something that triggered sleeplessness in the first place. The paradox is that if you are not prepared to accept the discomfort of your sleeplessness, you may never experience good quality sleep.

Case Study Continued . . . On realising how she had bought into her fears and allowed her life to become defined by fighting her insomnia, Patricia felt angry and upset. She could not believe how she had let the situation get so out of hand and had not noticed what was happening sooner. She described having the urge to fight even harder and, when she was not noticing, found her mind quietly beating herself up. I explained that everything she had done was perfectly normal and how it is easy to get stuck in the fight when your life feels threatened. She recognised that she had a choice as to how she behaved and that continuing to be angry would not help her to move forward and certainly would not help her to sleep naturally.

The turning point for her was when she realised that by gently beginning to live her life and starting to do all of the things she had put on hold, such as going out with friends, finding a boyfriend and getting another job, she would not only be living her life but also lessening her struggle with poor sleep. She would have to learn to accept the discomfort that comes with poor sleep, but she could choose to start living from that moment on.

Getting your Life Back

Insomniacs often say: 'If I could just get rid of my insomnia, then I could start living my life again'. Buying into such a thought could leave you waiting for a very long time or worse still never actually living your life. If you have felt like this try to describe what this other life would look like and what you would be doing differently compared to now?

How would your new life be if you didn't have to spend all of your energy controlling your sleep? Aim for more things of value than I just want to sleep, have more energy or be happy because while they may be true, they aren't concrete enough for you to take action on. Here are some of the common value driven answers I've been given:

- 'I would spend more intimate time with my partner'
- 'I would share the same bed as my partner'
- 'I would play with my children'
- 'I would be finding a partner to love and support'
- 'I would run, go to the gym and eat healthier food'
- 'I would spend more time socialising with friends'
- 'I would be pregnant and starting a family of my own'
- 'I would work hard for a promotion at work'
- 'I would focus on my studies so that I can pass my exams'
- 'I would be more involved in my local neighbourhood'
- 'I would attend more art galleries, theatre and cinema'

Once you have a few things to mind, ask yourself if you could do any of those things right now. The answer is probably 'yes', because in reality there is nothing stopping you from doing these activities. It is the power that you have given to your insomnia that makes you believe that you can't do them. It is true that insomnia is debilitating, however even during the dark times when you feel your lowest you can always choose to act in a way that moves your life towards things of value. The steps may not be the leaps that you wished for, but even small steps move you further forward than if you remain stuck struggling with your insomnia.

Taking Action

If you are serious about getting your life back then now is the time to take action. Think of what you can do in the next 24 hours that will bring you closer to what is important to you in life and then do it. Remember the more small acts the better!

Text a friend to meet up for coffee, take your partner out for a meal, go to the gym before work, share your bed with your partner, eat a healthy lunch, play with your children at the park, go to watch a film at the cinema, help out your neighbour, sign up to internet dating or enrol on a course. Aim to do at least one helpful act every day and keep a diary of everything that you do.

Taking action could be likened to knocking over that first domino and then watching the series of small acts that automatically follow. More than likely you've become very good at sleeping badly because you repeated bad habits. What you are about to do now is exactly the same, except this time your actions are helping you to re-live your life to the full and become a great sleeper.

'I have found that living by my values gives me something to hold on to. It gives me a sense of achievement when I have attended an event, which in

the past I might have had second thoughts about. Plus I have realised that the more I do, the more confident I feel. 'It's my life and I'm going to write the script!'
Fran, UK

Case Study Continued . . . One obstacle that Patricia noticed was how much insomnia had knocked her self-confidence. She described how she used to be so outgoing and always up for a challenge, but now she questioned her ability to perform even simple tasks. She felt conflicted because on the one hand she really wanted to get back to living her life and yet on the other doubted her ability to do it. I explained that many of my clients felt the same way. When you have spent a long period of time choosing to not live your life, you effectively get out of practice. Everyday events such as travelling to work, looking after children or meeting up with best friends can suddenly feel overwhelming. At this point it is easy to want to run away and escape again, but you know that this is not the answer.

Every day she chose to do things of importance and value, and found that the more she did, the easier it became. When I spoke to her a few months later, she said that her 'eureka' moment came when she recognised that her low self-confidence was just another passenger on her bus, and while she did not like it being there, she could decide whether to let it drive. From that point on she got on with her life and discovered that with each small thing she did, her self-confidence returned and her sleep improved.

'Failures are finger posts on the road to achievement.'
C.S. Lewis

When Insomnia Comes Back

If you've worked your way through this programme, you'll be starting to enjoy normal sleep again. Mentally you feel alert, focused, confident and even happy with life. Physically you feel light, energetic and ready to pounce on any physical challenge that comes your way. Life is pretty good, or at least a lot better than when you weren't sleeping. Whether you've been sleeping well for one night, one week or one month, you begin to think that you have cracked it and your sleepless nights are over.

Then one night you find yourself awake. Your mind starts to ask what you can do to fix it, in the hope of nipping it in the bud as soon as possible. You have tasted normal sleep again and are prepared to do anything to keep it. Out of desperation you start to struggle and escape the arrivals that start to show up. Your heart begins to pound, your stomach knots, anxiety creeps in, and your thinking mind starts to calculate what you stand to lose if poor sleep does return. It seems that your normal sleep is shattered and your insomnia is back. But hang on ... The truth is, just because you have learnt to sleep normally again does not mean you are immune from insomnia. Mind you, nor is a normal sleeper.

Case Study Continued ... Within a few months Patricia's sleep had improved immensely and she had started to live her life again. For this reason she decided to go on holiday, something that she been avoiding for many years as a way of trying to control her sleep. She went to America and had a great holiday with her friends. However, on her return, like most people, she experienced some jet lag, which caused her to be awake at night. The shock of lying in bed awake instantly brought a wave of sabotaging thoughts that told her that everything was going to return to how it used to be and, worst of all, triggered the old sensations of anxiety and panic. Obviously this was the last place she wanted to be and she soon became consumed by urges to control her sleep. I got a phone call early the next morning and she told me everything that had happened and how she just wanted to go back to where she was before she left. She explained to me how she had tried to use all of the tools I had taught her, but nothing had worked.

At this moment I knew Patricia had been hooked by the sleep sabotage that gets so many of my clients when poor sleep returns. I explained to her that what she was going through was quite normal and how the wakefulness associated with jet lag had triggered all of her old fears. When I asked her what she meant by 'nothing had worked', she realised that in her desperation to prevent poor sleep from returning, she had inadvertently started to use the tools she had learnt with me to try and control her insomnia again rather than accept it. The end result was she had spent the whole night expending huge amounts of energy struggling with her sleeplessness rather than just being awake because of jet lag. This experience highlighted to Patricia just how easy it is to start struggling with poor sleep again, especially when you think you have cracked it! It also showed her how deep down she still feared the presence of her insomnia and was unwilling to accept it into her life.

Your Brain Remembers Your Insomnia

Remember, your brain is a thinking machine that is constantly linking bits of information together and using them as a reference for anticipating what might happen in the present or the future. As we covered in Week 1, there is a cost of having such a brilliant problem-solving machine at your disposal. All you need to do is believe and act upon your mind's projected tales of sleeplessness and you can keep yourself awake for days. Understanding this process is not only paramount for learning how to sleep naturally again, we also need to remind ourselves of it to prevent a relapse.

Remember Week 1, in which we pointed out that almost everyone on the planet will experience a poor night or two at some point in their life? Triggers such as work issues, family arguments, financial worries, jet lag or even just the common cold can be enough to induce a short bout of sleeplessness. However, for the majority of people, once the stress is resolved, their sleep returns to its original pattern because the brain has no reason for it not to.

In the case of a recovering insomniac, this is not always true, because your thinking mind struggles to distinguish between what would be considered a normal night of poor sleep and the possible threat of insomnia returning. This means that while your returning bout of poor sleep will probably pass within a few days, your mind can't help but ask the inevitable question 'What if this is the start of my insomnia returning?' Once again this is not some sort of malicious act, but rather your mind accessing your chequered sleep history and using it to flag up any potential risks for the future.

> Your brain will always remember your poor sleep history and so you will always have a greater risk of experiencing poor sleep than someone who has never had insomnia.

Sometimes it only takes the suggestion of poor sleep for it to be triggered. For example, if your insomnia was originally triggered by events in your life such as work stress or pregnancy, experiencing them again is a possible trigger. Sometimes it can even be sleeping well that reminds you of sleeping badly and that triggers the return of poor sleep.

Ironically, I've had people cancel their Sleep School appointment to avoid having to think about poor sleep and potentially upset their so-called 'good run'. Sadly, as you know, what you resist persists and so if you go with your fear of poor sleep returning, you increase the likelihood that it will return.

How you choose to act when the thought or reality of a sleepless night crops up determines whether you amplify or reduce the possibility of chronic insomnia returning. If you feel worried about this, then revisit Weeks 2 and 3 to remind yourself of how to skilfully acknowledge it and yet not pay it enough attention to cause any unwanted amplification. Act like a normal sleeper and regard it as a one-off thing.

Before you feel that all is lost and that there is no point reading any further, remember just because you have past memories of poor sleep doesn't mean it's inevitable that you'll experience it again. Remember the example I gave earlier

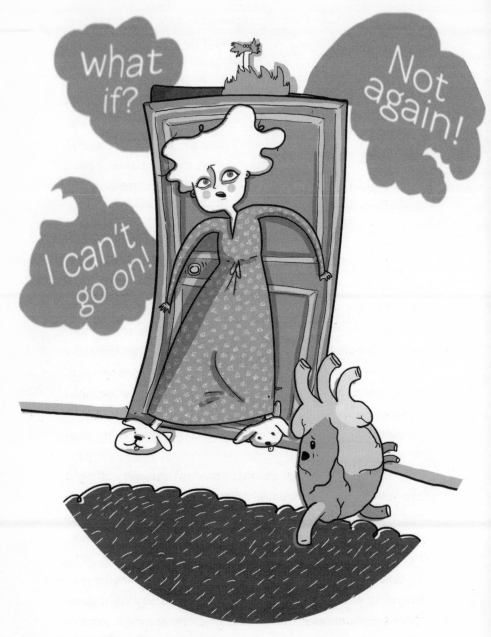

Fig. 5.3 The Return of Poor Sleep

showing that how a person behaves towards dogs after being bitten determines the power and longevity of the response. So if you chose to avoid all dogs in the future, you would have the short-term benefit of not feeling scared, but run the risk of the long-term consequence of always being afraid of dogs. In contrast, if you decided to make contact with dogs again and learnt that not all dogs are harmful, such fear can become almost non-existent over time. It's only by being open to the possibility of poor sleep returning that you can slip back into peaceful slumber.

Case Study Continued . . . Patricia described that as soon as the thought 'What if my poor sleep returns?' had popped into her head, it was like a door had opened in her body allowing every other unwanted guest to show up. Suddenly she had felt a pang of anxiety in her stomach, a quickening of her heart rate, a tightening of her muscles and an overwhelming urge to block them all. The more she tried to get rid of the feelings, the stronger they became and the more her mind catastrophised about how bad things were going to get. She mentioned feeling completely powerless against them and yet unable to stop herself from struggling.

On hearing how Patricia had battled with her sleep all night and sensing her continued frustration, I asked her to revisit the night in her mind. Except this time I wanted her to objectively describe out loud everything that showed up for her in order. I guided her search with descriptive questions such as 'Who showed up for you?', 'Where was all this happening in your body?', 'What were your emotions doing?' and so on. She knew these techniques well and had no problem slowing down and taking notice.

Afterwards she described the difference between what she had been doing and what she had just done. She could instantly see how in the heat of the moment everything she had done had been focused on the goal of getting rid of her insomnia and that there was very little acceptance. She was amazed at just how much she had bought into the sabotage and how her unwillingness to allow it in had led to her experience greater levels of panic, frustration and wakefulness once more. I explained to her that being open to experiencing the sabotage was a vital part of keeping her good sleep on track.

Taking Effective Action

Being calm and accepting of the occasional poor night's sleep is a key part to sleep maintenance and the last step to sleeping well. Insomniacs who achieve long-term recovery from their insomnia are those who are willing to let go of struggle and instead notice and accept their mind's and body's reactions to insomnia. They recognise that fighting insomnia is not only tiring but also futile. They understand that a bad night does not have to spell the return of their insomnia. If you have already had a recurrence of poor sleep and allowed it to mindfully pass, then congratulate yourself, as this is a fundamental part of your recovery. You are making progress. The more practised you are at noticing and letting go of your reactions to poor sleep when they arrive, the less power they have and the closer to a normal sleeper you become.

How you deal with the return of insomnia is exactly the same as how you have dealt with your insomnia so far. Here is a recap of the programme so you can easily find it when you need it.

Accepting

One of the most common reasons for insomnia returning is loss of awareness. When you start sleeping better and your life no longer revolves around getting to sleep, it is easy to let your noticing practice slip.

I frequently hear 'It was all going so well, so I thought I didn't need to practise.' You don't need to practise for hours every day, but a little bit of practice such as noticing your senses when you are walking down the street or noticing your breath can be enough to keep you from becoming stuck again. Everything that you have learnt in this book is about increasing your awareness of how you can get in the way of your sleep, not about controlling your sleep. Gentle practice helps you to notice your experiences as they unfold, helping you to choose how to respond to them, *not* to get in the way of your sleep.

The act of being mindful will become helpful in all areas of your life. For example, if you are having a conversation and you notice that your mind is off thinking about whether you will sleep tonight, you can return your attention to your discussion. Equally when you are in a meeting, at the gym, watching TV or at the theatre, you want to be present in order to fully experience what you are doing. If you are out of practice with the noticing exercises, then reread Week 2.

Welcoming

Welcoming allows you to create space for the thoughts, emotions, sensations and urges that show up inside you. It is characterised by being willing to experience, own and even play with them. In doing so, you send a powerful message to your brain that you are safe. As a result you feel less need to struggle to avoid, change or get rid of them and so wake yourself up less, save your valuable energy and can refocus your attention on living your life.

Building

There is no point building a house unless it has good foundations; equally there is no point working on improving your sleep unless you have built a strong sleeping pattern to help sleep flourish.

This means attending to the basics by making sure that the duration and timing of your sleep are correct for you. When you have a bad night's sleep, it can be easy to slip back into old unhelpful habits such as lying in bed late to catch up on sleep, despite the fact that you know it will weaken your drive for the next night and confuse your clock. If you are still unsure about your sleeping pattern, then look back at Week 4.

How to Behave like a Normal Sleeper

Remember, to become a normal sleeper you have to act like one:

- Accept that before you can get back to doing nothing, there's some work to do. I know it's frustrating, but I promise it will be worth it.
- Create a relaxed and flexible approach to sleep that treats it as an ordinary part of everyday life, rather than the pivot around which your world revolves.
- Let go of any unnecessary sleep props that you use.
- It is essential to learn to stay in bed and rest, rather than get up through the night.
- If you are going to create an environment for sleep to emerge, then it is important to achieve a balance in

these areas whereby you do enough to promote sleep and yet do not allow them to become a point of obsession.

- Don't give everything up – take a balanced approach to food and drink and going out at night.

Learning to Live

Now it's time to move on to the final stage of the Five-Week Programme: living. I've had insomniacs complete the programme who suddenly have a new lease of life, deciding to go for a promotion at work, start exercising regularly and enrol themselves on a university course. They feel fantastic because their life is finally heading in the direction they wanted it to. It is vital to remember, however, that your recovery is not a straight path. Unforeseen events will rise up and challenge you, and the odd sleepless night is one of them.

For other people, a blip in their sleeping confirms their original fears and they find themselves thinking, 'I knew this good run of sleep wouldn't last,' and that following their heart has made them vulnerable to the pain. To make things worse, they now feel they stand to lose much more and fall so much further than if they had just remained under their old faithful comfort blanket of avoidance.

At this point have the flexibility to briefly moderate your plans rather than give up on them altogether. This allows you to manage any sleeplessness skilfully and allow it to pass as quickly as it arrived. For example, this may mean choosing to go for a walk rather than a run, or choosing to call a friend rather than meet up. Either way, living your life in the way you want to ignites a natural sense of ease inside you, which is transferred to your sleep. You are much more likely to sleep if your brain knows the world around you is safe and secure.

I have worked with many insomniacs who have chosen to stop living their lives in order to try and fight their insomnia. In every case the fight has been futile and only led to the further development of their insomnia and the narrowing of their valuable life. Remember, you can't stop yourself from experiencing poor sleep, but you can determine how much it costs you and your life. By adopting a gentle, non-judging and accepting attitude towards it you weaken the power that it holds over you.

Take Action

As the saying goes, 'You can lead a horse to water, but you can't make it drink.' Throughout this programme we have revealed how your insomnia started, learnt to watch and welcome all of the unwanted arrivals in your mind and body, learnt how to build yourself a new sleeping pattern and now what you want your life to stand for. However, this will all be for nothing unless you decide to take action. You can follow your familiar path of control and avoidance, which may still appear attractive or safe despite not actually helping. Alternatively you can follow a new path of acceptance and commitment, whereby you willingly choose to accept your life as it is at this moment, with your insomnia, so that you can move boldly forward.

I wholeheartedly hope that you now feel equipped to make the commitment and take the steps to make this happen.

'I'd been following the Sleep School programme for about six months, with great success on the whole. Naturally, I thought I had "cracked it", although I didn't like to admit that too loudly, it was definitely a thought. Which was perfect as I had quite a stressful week-long work trip on the near horizon, followed by a special holiday, and of course I wanted to be at my best for both – which meant sleeping well.

As the time approached, the pressure piled up. The desire for sleep perfection, to protect what I'd so carefully cultivated, surfaced. As the inevitable downward spiral began and my sleep unravelled, all the tools came out of the box! Increasingly, I tried them all out – at times I felt like I was firefighting in the middle of the night using one tool after another in a desperate bid to control the sleep. All the while, completely losing sight of their true purpose. This was nothing new, it just felt like a new situation because it was a relapse.

The impatient urge to "fix it" was still there, until I hit the bottom, and was smacked around the face with the reality that it's a fight you will never win and the only way is to let go! Eventually, I was able to step back and see the situation for what it was and begin slowly practising the "not doing" once again'.

Christine, London

Onward Journey

On finishing the Sleep School Programme, people often comment that they have the properties of an insomniac but now sleep well. This tells me a lot about their progress because it means that they accept the fact that they have insomnia in their memory bank, but recognise that it needn't determine the way they sleep and live their life. They have responded to any ongoing sabotage in such a skilful manner as to teach their brain that they are no longer under attack and that it is okay for natural sleep to emerge. Repetition of the process reduces the power and frequency of insomnia recurrence until it fades away.

If you would like to see how far you have come, then go back to the Introduction and look at your 'Sleep School Insomnia Survey'. If you would like to fill it out again, then do so at the www.thesleepschool.org

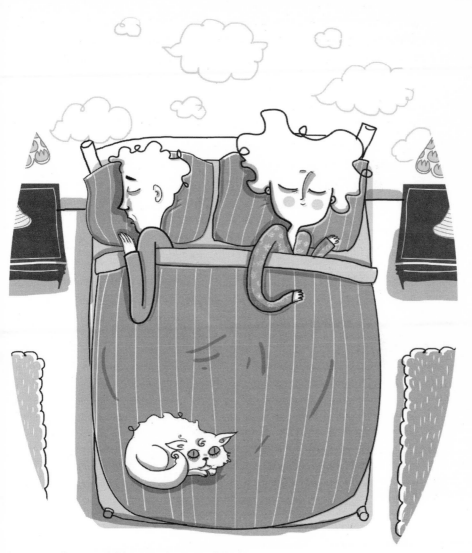

Fig. 5.3 **Wishing You the Best of Sleep**

Conclusion

'I used to think my brain was the most important organ – until I noticed which organ was telling me that'

Emo Philips

Congratulations. I hope you've come a long way with your sleep and are now resting and sleeping more easily. No doubt it hasn't been the easiest journey that you've ever taken, but it could quite possibly be the best, because there is nothing like waking up after a fantastic night's sleep.

During this programme you'll have discovered that struggling to control your sleep simply kept you awake. By accepting and taking note of what shows up in your mind and body at night and when necessary welcoming it, even when all you want to do is fight it, you'll have regained some of your energy and zest for life.

If you've followed the programme, you'll have built a new sleeping pattern that naturally drives you into peaceful slumber. And finally you have learnt to start living your life more fully again. Working your way through this book, practising mindfulness and acceptance, will have indirectly, rather than forcefully, moved you and your body closer towards sleep.

Mindfully accepting slows you down; welcoming implies safety; building creates strong foundations; and living creates contentment. All of which promote fantastic sleep.

Your job now is to get on and live your life as a normal sleeper. If you have the occasional poor night's sleep, that just means you are now a normal sleeper again, and one night needn't hail the return of chronic insomnia!

If you do find yourself lying awake again, relax and accept it, and remind yourself of the steps you've taken over these past weeks. Practise any parts of the programme that you think could help you.

Here's a checklist to make sure you've covered the key steps:

Week 1. Discover and understand why you have insomnia in the first place by getting to know your risks, triggers, arrivals and amplifiers.

Week 2. The first step to having more energy is to stop struggling, let go and simply rest. Remain in the present and accept things as they are.

Week 3. Harness the power of the welcome response by inviting in all that shows up in your mind and body.

Week 4. Behave like a normal sleeper and build a healthy sleep-wake cycle.

Week 5. Keep your focus on living and you'll sleep better. Keep up your practice so that you can get back on track if insomnia tries to creep back in.

If you complete each Week of the book, the effects will be strong and lasting, both for your sleep and the rest of your life.

If, like many others who've completed this programme, you're back to sleeping well, then enjoy it – lie back and do nothing, just like a normal sleeper.

Wishing you a long and happy life of good sleep.

You've earned it.

Dr. Guy Meadows

Appendix

Additional Support and Information
Support
Free Sleep School Worksheets
To assist your journey through this book, you can download a variety of free worksheets, info sheets and audio tracks from www.thesleepschool.org.

The Sleep School App
To receive additional support, you can download The Sleep School app by going to www.thesleepschool.org. This programme takes you through the The Sleep School's Five-Week programme with the use of supportive tools, mindfulness tracks, educational animations, and audio and video content that is not included in the book.

The Sleep School Classes
If you would be interested in attending one of the courses, workshops or retreats please visit www.thesleepschool.org to find out about future dates.

Books on Acceptance and Commitment Therapy
Steven C. Hayes and Spencer Smith, *Get Out of Your Mind and Into Your Life: The New Acceptance and Commitment Therapy*, New Harbinger Publications, Oakland, California, 2005

Useful Web Links

To learn more about Acceptance and Commitment Therapy please visit www.contextualscience.org.

Or watch the acceptance and commitment therapy 'Animated Metaphors' by Joe Oliver entitled 'Unwelcome Party Guest', 'Demons on the Boat' and 'Passengers on the Bus'.

Endnotes

[1] Hayes, S. C., Strosahl, K. D., and Wilson, K. G. (1999). *Acceptance and commitment therapy: An experiential approach to behavior change.* New York: Guilford Press.

[2] Spielman, A., and Glovinsky, P. (1991). The varied nature of insomnia. In P. Hauri (Ed.). *Case studies in insomnia.* New York: Plenum.

[3] Burch Vidyamala, (2008). *Living Well With Chronic Pain and Illness: The Mindful Way to Free Yourself From Suffering.* London: Piatkus.

[4] Gross C.R. *et al.*, Mindfulness-based stress reduction versus pharmacotherapy for chronic primary insomnia: a randomised controlled clinical trial. *Explore,* New York, 2011, 7 (2): 76–87.

[5] Hölzel, B.K. *et al.*, (2011). Mindfulness practice leads to increases in regional brain gray matter density. *Psychiatry Res.* 30;191(1):36-43.

[6] Gold, D. B. and Wegner, D. M. Origins of ruminative thought: trauma, incompleteness, nondisclosure, and suppression, *Journal of Applied Social Psychology,* 1995, 25: 1245–61.

[7] Yoo, S.S. *et al.*, The human emotional brain without sleep: a prefrontal-amygdala disconnect, *Current Biology,* 2007, 17 (20): 877–8.

[8] Walker, M. P. and Stickgold, R. Sleep, memory and plasticity, *Annual Review of Psychology,* 2006, 57: 139–66.

[9] Breslau, N. *et al.*, Sleep disturbance and psychiatric disorders: a longitudinal epidemiological study of young adults.

Biol Psychiatry, 1996, (39): 411–418.

[10] Lieberman, M. D. *et al.*, Putting feelings into words: affect labeling disrupts amygdala activity in response to affective stimuli. *Psychological Science,* 2007, 18 (5): 421–8.

Index